THE
ENDOCRINES

ATLAS *of* TUMOR RADIOLOGY

[10]

PHILIP J. HODES, M.D., *Editor-in-Chief*

Sponsored by

THE AMERICAN COLLEGE OF RADIOLOGY

—*with the cooperation of:*

AMERICAN CANCER SOCIETY
AMERICAN ROENTGEN RAY SOCIETY
CANCER CONTROL PROGRAM, USPHS
EASTMAN KODAK COMPANY
JAMES PICKER FOUNDATION
RADIOLOGICAL SOCIETY OF NORTH AMERICA

THE
ENDOCRINES

by

HOWARD L. STEINBACH, M.D.

Chief of Diagnostic Radiology, French Hospital, San Francisco;
Clinical Professor of Radiology, University of California, San Francisco Medical Center,
and Stanford University, Palo Alto, Calif.

and

HIDEYO MINAGI, M.D.

Assistant Professor of Radiology, Department of Radiology, University of California,
San Francisco Medical Center, and Assistant Radiologist,
San Francisco General Hospital

YEAR BOOK MEDICAL PUBLISHERS · INC.
35 EAST WACKER DRIVE, CHICAGO

Dedication to

ILSE, KATHY, LYNNE, LISA, CARYN, *and* XERO

Editor's Preface

In 1960, the Committee on Radiology of the National Research Council began to consider the preparation of a tumor atlas for radiology similar in concept to the Armed Forces Institute of Pathology's "Atlas of Tumor Pathology." So successfully had the latter filled a need in pathology that it seemed reasonable to establish a similar resource for radiology. Therefore a subcommittee of the Committee on Radiology was appointed to study the concept and make recommendations.

That original committee, made up of Dr. Russell H. Morgan (Chairman), Dr. Marshall H. Brucer and Dr. Eugene P. Pendergrass, reported that a need did indeed exist and recommended that something be done about it. That report was unanimously accepted by the parent committee.

Soon thereafter, there occurred a normal change of the membership of the Committee on Radiology of the Council. This was followed by a change of the "Atlas" subcommittee, which now included Dr. E. Richard King (Chairman), Dr. Leo G. Rigler and Dr. Barton R. Young. To this new subcommittee was assigned the task of finding how the "Atlas" was to be published. Numerous avenues were explored; none seemed wholly satisfactory.

With the passing of time, it became increasingly apparent that the American College of Radiology had to be brought into the picture. It had prime teaching responsibilities; it had a Commission on Education; it seemed the logical responsible agent to launch the "Atlas." Confident of the merits of this approach, the entire Committee on Radiology of the Council became involved in focusing the attention of the American College of Radiology upon the matter.* In 1964, as the result of their persuasiveness, the Board of Chancellors of the American College of Radiology named an ad hoc committee to explore and define the scholarly scope of the "Atlas" and the probable costs. In 1965, the ad hoc committee recommended that the College

---

* At that time, the Committee on Radiology included, in addition to the subcommittee, Drs. John A. Campbell, James B. Dealy, Jr., Melvin M. Figley, Hymer L. Friedell, Howard B. Latourette, Alexander Margulis, Ernest A. Mendelsohn, Charles M. Nice, Jr., and Edward W. Webster.

sponsor and publish the "Atlas." Accordingly, an Editorial Advisory Committee was chosen to work within the Commission on Education with authority to select an Editor-in-Chief. At the same time, the College provided funds for starting the project and began representations for grants-in-aid without which the "Atlas" would never be published.

No history of the "Atlas of Tumor Radiology" would be complete without specific recording of the generous response of the several radiological societies, as well as the private and Federal granting institutions whose names appear on the title page and below among our acknowledgments. It was their tangible evidence of confidence in the project that provided everyone with enthusiasm and eagerness to achieve our goal.

The "Atlas of Tumor Radiology" includes all major organ systems. It is intended to be a systematic body of pictorial and written information dealing with the roentgen manifestations of tumors. No attempt has been made to provide an atlas equivalent of a medical encyclopedia. Nevertheless the "Atlas" is designed to serve as an important reference source and teaching file for all physicians, not radiologists alone.

The twelve volumes of the "Atlas," to be completed in 1971-72, are: *The Hemopoietic and Lymphatic Systems,* by Gerald D. Dodd and Sidney Wallace; *The Bones and Joints,* by Gwilym Lodwick and Lent C. Johnson; *The Lower Respiratory Tract and Thoracic Contents,* by Roy R. Greening and J. Haynes Heslep; *The Gastrointestinal Tract,* by Arthur K. Finkelstein and George N. Stein; *The Urinary Tract,* by John A. Evans and Morton Bosniak; *The Breast,* by David M. Witten; *The Head and Neck,* by Gilbert H. Fletcher and Bao-Shan Jing; *The Nervous System and the Eye,* by Juan M. Taveras and Ernest W. Wood; *The Female Generative System,* by G. Melvin Stevens and John F. Weigen; *The Endocrines,* by Howard L. Steinbach and Hideyo Minagi; *The Accessory Digestive Organs,* by Robert E. Wise; and *The Spine,* by Bernard S. Epstein.

Some overlapping of material in several volumes is inevitable, for example, tumors of the female generative system, tumors of the endocrine glands and tumors of the urinary tract. This is considered to be an asset. It assures the specialist completeness in the volume or volumes that concern him and provides added breadth and depth of knowledge for those interested in the entire series.

The broad scope of the "Atlas of Tumor Radiology" has precluded its preparation by a single or even several authors. To maintain uniformity of format, rather rigid criteria were established early. These included manner of presentation, size of illustrations, as well as style of headings, subheadings and legends. The authors were encouraged to keep the text at a minimum, freeing as much space as possible for large illustrations and meaningful legends. The "Atlas" is to be just that, an "atlas," not a series of "texts." The authors were urged, also, to keep the bibliography brief.

The selection of suitable authors for the "Atlas" was extremely difficult, and to a degree invidious. For the final choice, the Editor-in-Chief accepts full responsibility. It is but fair to record, however, that his Editorial Advisory Committee accepted his recommendations. The format of the "Atlas," too, was the choice of the Editor-in-Chief, again with the concurrence of his advisory group. Should the "Atlas of Tumor Radiology" fall short of its goals, the fault will lie with the Editor-in-Chief alone; his Editorial Advisory Committee was selfless in its dedication to the purposes of the "Atlas," rendering invaluable advice and guidance whenever asked to do so.

As medical knowledge expands, medical concepts change. In medicine, the written word considered true today may not be so tomorrow. The text of the "Atlas," considered true today, therefore may not be true tomorrow. What may not change, what may ever remain true, may be the illustrations of the "Atlas of Tumor Radiology." Their legends may change as our conceptual levels advance. But the validity of the roentgen findings there recorded should endure. Thus, if the fidelity with which the roentgenograms have been reproduced is of superior order, the illustrations in the "Atlas" should long serve as sources for reference no matter what revisions of the text become necessary with advancing medical knowledge.

ACKNOWLEDGMENTS

The American College of Radiology, its Commission on Education, the Editorial Advisory Committee, the authors and the Editor-in-Chief wish to acknowledge their grateful appreciation:

1. For the grants-in-aid so willingly and repeatedly provided by The American Cancer Society, The American Roentgen Ray Society, The Cancer Control Program, National Center for Chronic Disease Control (USPHS Grant No. 59481), The James Picker Foundation, and The Radiological Society of North America.

2. For the superb glossy print reproductions provided by the Radiography Markets Division, Eastman Kodak Company. Special mention must be made of the sustained interest of Mr. George R. Struck, its Assistant Vice-President and General Manager. We applaud particularly Mr. William

S. Cornwell, Technical Associate and Editor Emeritus of Kodak's *Medical Radiography and Photography,* as well as his associates, Mr. Charles C. Heckman and Mr. Stanley J. Pietrzkowski and others in the Photo Service Division, whose expertise provided the "Atlas" with its incomparable photographic reproductions.

3. To Year Book Medical Publishers, for their personal involvement with and judicious guidance in the many problems of publication. There were occasions when the publisher questioned the quality of certain illustrations. Almost always the judgment of the authors and the Editor-in-Chief prevailed because of the importance of the original roentgenograms and the singular fidelity of their reproduction.

4. To the Associate Editors, particularly Mrs. Anabel I. Janssen, whose talents lightened the burden of the Editor-in-Chief and helped establish the style of presentation of the material.

5. To the Staff of the American College of Radiology, especially Messrs. William C. Stronach, Otha Linton, Keith Gundlach and William Melton, for continued conceptual and administrative efforts of unusual competence.

One of the difficulties that faced our present authors concerned the inclusion in their volume of the pineal, hypothalamus, and testicle. Strictly speaking, these are not endocrine glands; yet their humoral potentiating effects seemed to require that they be presented. Despite the added load this imposed upon Dr. Steinbach and Dr. Minagi, they cheerfully agreed to include them. For this and especially for the rapid and selfless manner in which they went about completing their task, we are deeply grateful. The authors, appreciating the need for radiographic excellence, never hesitated to set aside their own roentgen studies for others that might have been but slightly superior. This was particularly true of tumors of less common occurrence in the pancreas and adrenal.

For obvious reasons, *The Endocrines* deals with tumors that will be included in other volumes of the "Atlas." This the authors knew and were encouraged to ignore.

The "Atlas of Tumor Radiology" is being published in a time when massive scientific effort is taking place at an unprecedented rate and on an unprecedented scale. We hope that our final product will provide an authoritative summary of our current knowledge of the roentgen manifestations of tumors.

PHILIP J. HODES

Jefferson Medical College   *Editor-in-Chief*

Editorial Advisory Committee

HARRY L. BERMAN   VINCENT P. COLLINS   E. RICHARD KING

LEO G. RIGLER   PHILIP RUBIN

Author's Preface

THIS volume represents an attempt to present in a succinct form the important roentgen features of tumors and tumor-like lesions affecting the many endocrine glands. The changes seen on plain roentgenograms have been emphasized and, when applicable, contrast examinations including angiographic and pneumographic have been described and illustrated.

The task was complicated by the rapid progress and changing concepts of endocrine glands and their secretions. Tumors of some regions, such as the hypothalamus, were included because at the time this volume was being compiled, the prevailing opinion of most experts in the field indicated that these lesions either secreted hormones or influenced the secretion of hormones by other endocrines.

In each chapter we have included pertinent clinical, laboratory and pathologic data as well as descriptions of the roentgenographic appearance of the lesions and their metastatic neoplasms. The usual appearance, as well as variations, are described.

This volume would not have been completed were it not for the gentle persuasion, persistence and great helpfulness of Dr. Philip J. Hodes. Members of the Department of Radiology of the University of California and the San Francisco Medical Center have contributed cases. In particular, Dr. Thomas H. Newton and Dr. Alphonse Palubinskas have provided us with many illustrations of angiograms and pneumograms. Dr. Frank Zboralske of Stanford University, Dr. Stewart Reuter of Wayne County General Hospital, Eloise, Mich., Dr. Marcia Bilbao of the University of Oregon, and the late Dr. John Hope of Children's Hospital of Philadelphia have also contributed roentgenograms that have enhanced the value of this presentation.

HOWARD L. STEINBACH
HIDEYO MINAGI

PART 1

The Pituitary

Characteristics of Pituitary Tumors
and Acromegaly

CHROMOPHOBE ADENOMA

CHROMOPHOBE ADENOMA, a tumor of adulthood, comprises about 7% of all brain tumors and between 60 and 95% of pituitary tumors. The incidence reaches a peak between age 31 and 50 years. No sex predilection has been noted.

PATHOLOGIC CHANGES.—The tumors may vary in size from microscopic foci to massive lesions that have profound direct pressure effects on neighboring structures. As a rule, larger adenomas are associated with gross expansion of the sella turcica inferiorly and in the anteroposterior diameter. Horizontal expansion is common, with encroachment on one or both cavernous sinuses. Possibly depending on the laxity of the diaphragma sellae, the tumors may or may not extend above the confines of the sella turcica.

Histologically, the cytoplasm of the tumor cells is finely granular and its affinity to any stain is weak. In this sense, these cells are "chromophobe."

CLINICAL FINDINGS.—Symptoms caused by chromophobe adenomas are the result of pressure on contiguous structures. Headache and visual disturbances are by far the most common manifestations. Because the optic chiasm lies directly above the diaphragma sellae, bitemporal hemianopsia is the most frequent visual defect. Loss of the visual field may not be symmetrical, however, because of asymmetrical tumor growth or anterior or posterior position of the chiasm.

Constitutional symptoms of pituitary insufficiency may be produced by compression of the surrounding normal glandular tissue; however, impaired vision is usually apparent before much evidence of pituitary insufficiency is noted. Hypogonadism is common in these patients. In females, it is manifested predominantly by amenorrhea. In males, loss of libido and potency and decrease of facial and body hair may be noted. Thyroid and adrenal dysfunction are slower to appear.

Chromophobe adenomas have been regarded traditionally as nonfunctioning tumors; however, evidence has indicated that Cushing's syndrome, acromegaly, thyrotoxicosis and perhaps galactorrhea may occur with what appear to be chromophobe adenomas.[1]

---

[1] Danowski, T. S.: *Clinical Endocrinology* (Baltimore: Williams & Wilkins Company, 1962), Vol. 1.

ROENTGEN CHANGES.—Except with minute tumors found incidentally at autopsy, enlargement of the sella turcica has been noted in 95% of chromophobe adenomas.[2] Larger tumors may completely destroy the posterior clinoids and dorsum sellae, as well as erode the anterior clinoids (Fig. 1, *A*). An asymmetrical or central depression of the sellar floor by tumor often results in a "double-floored sella," as seen on the lateral view (Fig. 1, *B*). The dural roof of the hypophyseal fossa—the diaphragma sellae—is probably an important factor in limiting upward extension of pituitary tumors. Thus in a patient with a relatively tough sellar diaphragm, upward growth will be prevented until there has been considerable ballooning of the sella turcica. When the sellar diaphragm is relatively lax, however, the tumor may extend suprasellarly before much sellar enlargement has taken place.

Carotid arteriography is perhaps the most accurate means of delineating the lateral extension of the tumor (Figs. 3 and 4). This examination demonstrates the lateral displacement of the internal carotid arteries as they traverse the cavernous sinuses. Upward displacement of the anterior cerebral artery may also be appreciated (Fig. 3, *B*). Arteriography is most vital, however, in differentiating a pituitary tumor from an aneurysm of the internal carotid artery. Large aneurysms may give rise to sellar enlargement and clinical findings that are indistinguishable from those of chromophobe adenoma. An enlarged meningohypophyseal branch of the internal carotid artery supplying the tumor is occasionally demonstrated on carotid arteriograms.

Pneumoencephalography is the most reliable means of delimiting suprasellar extension of chromophobe adenomas (Fig. 2). Suprasellar extension may be limited to a slight bulge in the chiasmatic cistern, or it may be massive, displacing the third ventricle backward and spreading the anterior horns of the lateral ventricle. Occasionally, the tumor may grow upward sufficiently to obstruct the foramen of Monro. Rarely is lateral extension of the tumor sufficient to displace the temporal horns.

PITUITARY TUMORS MANIFESTED AFTER ADRENALECTOMY FOR CUSHING'S SYNDROME

Recent reports have indicated a significant incidence of pituitary tumors manifested after bilateral adrenalectomy for Cushing's syndrome secondary to adrenal hyperplasia (Fig. 6). Most of these have been diagnosed after adrenalectomy as chromophobe adenomas. Clinically, the presence of such tumors is suggested by development of abnormal pigmentation of skin, despite adequate replacement therapy after adrenalectomy. The tumors may grow

---

[2] Sheline, G. E.; Boldrey, E. B., and Phillips, T. L.: Chromophobe adenoma of the pituitary gland, Am. J. Roentgenol. 92:160, April, 1964.

rapidly and frequently are more aggressive than most pituitary neoplasms. Visual field loss in these patients develops and progresses rapidly. At times, the rapid growth of the tumor may be readily appreciated on serial roentgenograms of the skull.

BASOPHILIC ADENOMA

In contrast to the chromophobic and eosinophilic pituitary tumors that affect both sexes equally, the incidence of basophilic adenomas is some five times greater in females.[3] Basophilic tumors seldom give roentgenographic evidence of sellar enlargement, also in contrast to the chromophobe and eosinophilic adenomas. The clinical and roentgenographic features of pituitary basophilism are the result of adrenocortical hyperfunction and are described in Section 5, on adrenal tumors.

Evidence of sellar enlargement and extrasellar extension of a tumor may be seen occasionally with basophilic adenoma when the tumor becomes manifest after adrenalectomy.

ACROMEGALY

Acromegaly is a chronic disease characterized by enlargement of the bones, cartilage and soft tissues of the entire body induced by excessive secretion of growth hormone.

PATHOLOGIC CHANGES.—An increase in size and function of a portion of the anterior lobe of the pituitary gland has been well established as the cause of the disease. The lesion of the pituitary gland has been regarded generally as an eosinophilic adenoma or, occasionally, a hyperplasia of the eosinophilic cells without adenomatous formation. In many instances, however, the pituitary tumors associated with acromegaly have been composed of cells histologically indistinguishable from those of the chromophobe adenoma.[4]

In most series, eosinophilic adenomas comprise 5–30% of all pituitary tumors.[5] No sex predilection has been noted.

Thickening of the skin, resulting in coarsening of the features and accentuation of the folds of the skin and scalp, results primarily from increased connective tissue. The hair follicles, sebaceous glands and sweat glands, however, also increase in size and number. Hyperplasia of connective tissue has been noted in the supporting network of the bronchi, the periportal connec-

---

[3] Danowski: *Op. cit.*

[4] Young, D. G.; Bahn, R. C., and Randall, R. V.: Pituitary tumors associated with acromegaly, J. Clin. Endocrinol. 25:249, February, 1965.

[5] Danowski: *Op. cit.*

tive tissue of the liver and the interstitial tissue of the pancreas, heart and other organs. The joints are enlarged by thickening of the synovia, bursas, cartilage, ligaments, capsule and bone, accompanied by intra-articular fusion.

When endochondral and appositional bone growth is accelerated because of excretion of abnormal amounts of growth hormone before fusion of the epiphysis to the metaphysis, gigantism results. Since in most cases acromegaly begins during puberty or later, height increases little, if any. Under the stimulus of abnormal amounts of growth hormone, however, endochondral bone growth is still possible at specific sites. Thus cartilaginous proliferation and subsequent ossification at the mandibular condyle may produce an elongated mandible. Such proliferation and ossification may also be demonstrated in the ribs at the costochondral junction, resulting in a large chest cavity.

The accelerated appositional bone growth in acromegaly is accompanied by excessive bone resorption in some regions of the skeleton, such as the paranasal sinuses (Fig. 9, *B*) and short tubular bones. Osteoporosis is also a reflection of excessive bone resorption, but is not a constant finding in acromegaly.

ROENTGEN CHANGES.—Roentgenographically demonstrable changes of acromegaly are the result of excessive secretion of growth hormone. They may be reflected in abnormalities of bone, cartilage and soft tissue. Any or all of the recognized pathologic alterations of acromegaly may be missing on roentgenograms. The roentgenographic manifestations of acromegaly are the result of both the endocrine effect of the hypersecreting adenoma and the mechanical effect of local tumor growth.

The most consistent manifestation of local tumor growth is enlargement of the sella turcica (Figs. 7–10). It may be noted in as many as 90% of acromegalic patients.[6] The sellar configuration is of little value in differentiating eosinophilic tumors from chromophobe adenomas. Pneumoencephalographic and arteriographic manifestations of local tumor growth depend on extrasellar extension of the eosinophilic tumor and are identical to those of chromophobe adenomas, described earlier.

Infrequently, the tumor will erode the sellar floor to extend inferiorly into the sphenoid sinus. When such an erosion is associated with acromegaly, an eosinophilic adenocarcinoma should be suspected, although benign neoplasms may act similarly.

The roentgenographically observed changes of acromegaly that result

---

[6] Lang, E. K.: Roentgenologic features of acromegaly, Am. J. Roentgenol. 86:321, August, 1961.

from excessive secretion of growth hormone may be found virtually throughout the body.

On roentgenograms of the skull, common findings in acromegaly are: an abnormally thick calvarium (Fig. 8); excessive development of the frontal sinuses (Figs. 7, 9 and 10); excessive aeration and development of the mastoids; elongation of the mandible with prognathism and an increase of the mandibular angle (Fig. 10); spreading of the teeth (Fig. 10); an abnormally large tongue, and overgrowth of the external occipital protuberance. These changes are largely the result of soft tissue hypertrophy and excessive resorption and apposition of bone. The spreading of the teeth may be a mechanical effect of the prognathism. Because of elongation of the mandible, the lower teeth overlap the upper. The upper teeth then come in contact with the interlingual surface of the lower, mechanically forcing the teeth outward and increasing the interdental spaces.

Extracranial overgrowth may be reflected in excessive development of the terminal tufts of the distal phalanges (Figs. 11 and 12). Hyperostosis at the sites of ligamentous insertions is frequent. Vertebral hyperostosis, especially marked on the anterior aspect of the bodies, is often present and produces a large anteroposterior diameter (Fig. 14).

Abnormal proliferation of cartilage is manifested by excessive widening of joint spaces, particularly in the hands and feet (Figs. 11 and 12). The joints of acromegalic patients are prone to early and severe degenerative changes (Fig. 13).

A large tongue, seen on lateral skull roentgenograms (Fig. 10), may be a manifestation of soft tissue hypertrophy and visceromegaly. Corrugated soft tissue furrows may be observed overlying the posterior neck and occiput. Unusually thick subcalcaneal soft tissues are consistently noted on lateral roentgenograms of the feet.

Excessive bone resorption is often manifested by the presence of abnormally thin bones, particularly the metatarsals and proximal phalanges of the feet. The metacarpals and bones of the pubic wing may also be abnormally thin.

Figure 1.—Sella turcica changes in chromophobe adenoma.

A, lateral view. The sella turcica is expanded, with thinning of the dorsum sellae (**a**), erosion of one anterior clinoid (**b**) and depression of the sellar floor (**c**).

B, lateral view. The sella turcica is enlarged, with marked thinning of the dorsum sella (**a**). The sellar floor is disrupted (**c**), and there is slight intrasphenoid extension of tumor (**arrows**).

C, lateral tomogram. The dorsum sellae has been destroyed. Shell-like calcification is present around the periphery of the tumor (**arrows**).

D, oblique view. Erosion of the sphenoid strut. With anterior and lateral extension of the tumor, the bony strut separating the optic foramen and superior orbital fissure has been destroyed, resulting in a single large defect (**d**).

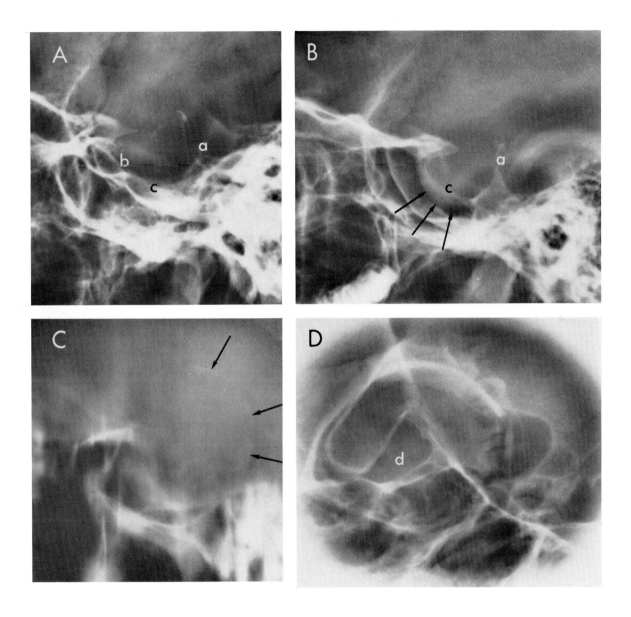

Figure 1 · Chromophobe Adenoma: Sella Turcica / 9

Figure 2.—Pneumoencephalographic changes in chromophobe adenoma.

A, lateral pneumoencephalogram. Suprasellar extension of the tumor is outlined by gas in the chiasmatic (**a**) and interpeduncular (**b**) cisterns.

B, lateral tomogram during pneumoencephalography. The suprasellar portion of the tumor (**arrows**) has caused upward and posterior displacement of the anterior portion of the third ventricle (**c**).

C, frontal tomogram during pneumoencephalography. The suprasellar portion of tumor is outlined by air (**solid arrows**). The basilar artery is also demonstrated (**open arrow**), as are the internal auditory meatuses (**d**).

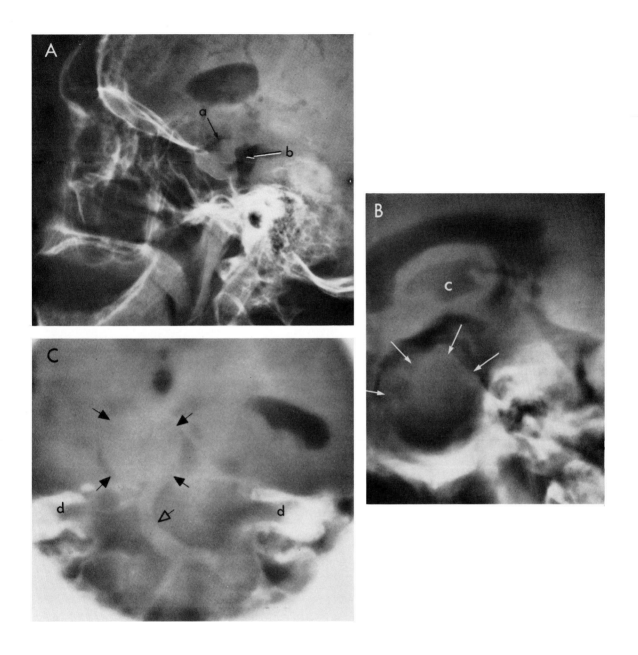

Figure 2 · Chromophobe Adenoma: Pneumoencephalography / 11

Figure 3.—Arteriographic changes in chromophobe adenoma.

A, internal carotid arteriogram, lateral view. The curve of the carotid siphon is widened (**a**) by suprasellar extension of the tumor. An enlarged meningohypophyseal trunk (**arrow**) supplies the tumor.

B, right and **C,** left carotid arteriograms, frontal views. The right anterior cerebral artery (**a**) is markedly elevated, whereas the left one (**b**) is in normal position. The tumor has extended into the suprasellar area predominantly on the right side.

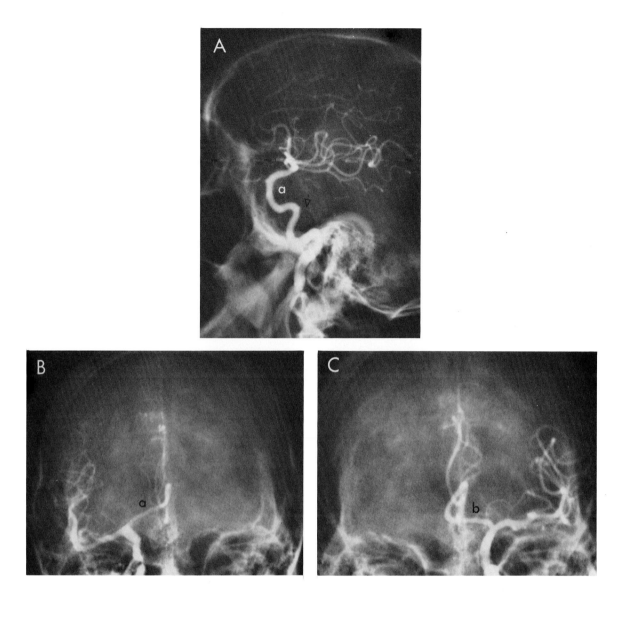

Figure 3 · Chromophobe Adenoma: Arteriography / 13

Figure 4.—Arteriographic changes in chromophobe adenoma.

A, internal carotid arteriogram, lateral view. During the venous phase, upward displacement of the basal vein is demonstrated (**arrows**), a manifestation of suprasellar extension of the tumor.

B, vertebral arteriogram, lateral view. Suprasellar extension of tumor has displaced the basilar artery posteriorly (**arrows**).

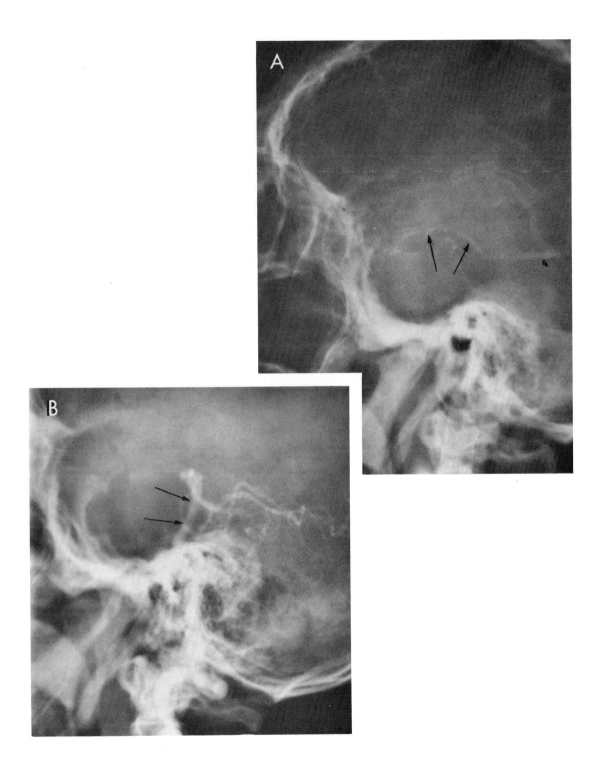

Figure 4 · Chromophobe Adenoma: Arteriography / 15

Figure 5.—Slipped epiphyses with chromophobe adenoma.

A, anteroposterior roentgenogram. The ossification centers for the femoral heads, normally fused by aged 18, are not fused in this patient at age 21.

B, anteroposterior roentgenogram. At age 23, both femoral capital epiphyses have slipped.

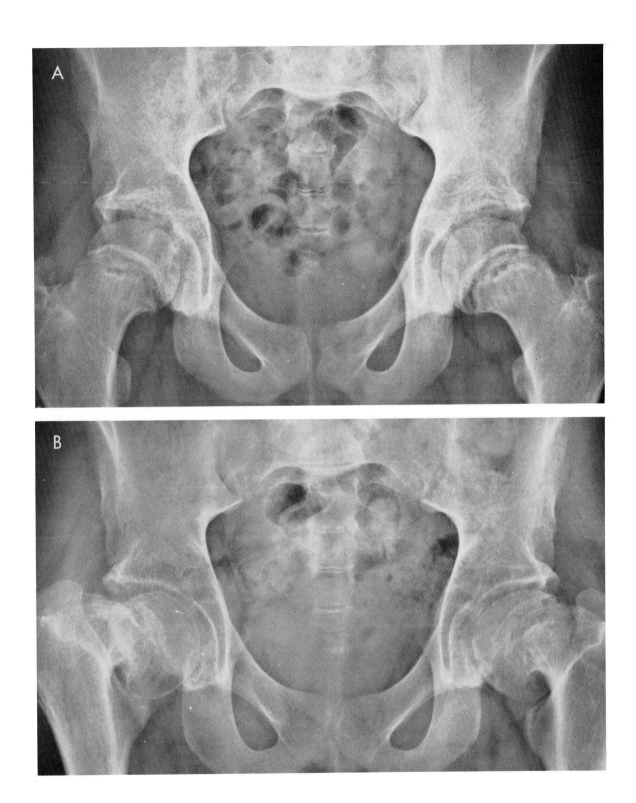

Figure 5 · Chromophobe Adenoma: Slipped Epiphyses / 17

Figure 6.—Pituitary tumors found after adrenalectomy for Cushing's syndrome.

A, lateral view: At the time of adrenalectomy for Cushing's syndrome. The sella turcica is of normal size.

B, lateral view: Seven years later. The sella turcica is elongated, with a double floor (**a**), and there is thinning of the dorsum sellae (**b**).

C, lateral view: At the time of adrenalectomy for Cushing's syndrome. The sella turcica is of normal size and configuration.

D, lateral view: Five years later. The sella turcica is enlarged, with a double floor (**a**) and thinning of the dorsum sellae (**b**).

Histologically, the tumor was a basophilic adenoma.

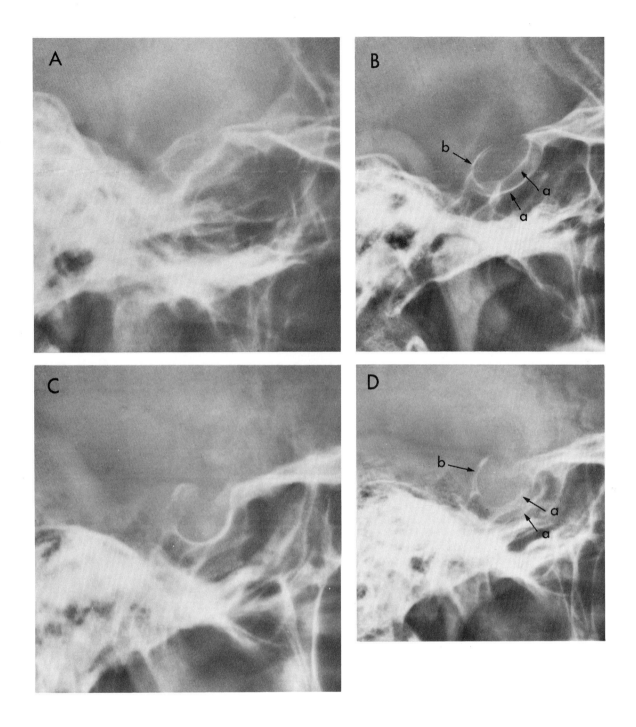

Figure 6 · Tumors after Adrenalectomy / 19

Figure 7.—Skull changes with acromegaly.

A, lateral view. The sella turcica (**a**) is enlarged, and there is unusual prominence of the frontal sinus (**b**). There is hyperostosis of the external occipital protuberance (**c**). The sellar configuration is of the so-called closed type.

B, lateral view. The sella turcica (**a**) is enlarged and the calvarium (**d**) thickened. Note the more open configuration of the sella in this patient.

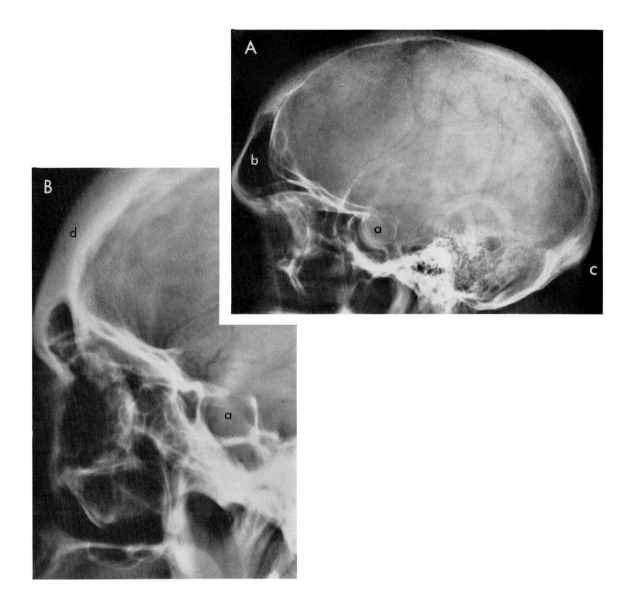

Figure 7 · Acromegaly: Skull Changes / 21

Figure 8.—Skull changes with acromegaly.

A, lateral view. The size and configuration of the sella turcica are normal (**a**); however, the calvarium is slightly thickened (**d**).

B, lateral view. There is enlargement of the sella turcica with destruction of its floor (**a**). The calvarium is markedly thickened (**d**).

C, lateral view. The sella turcica is enlarged, and there is calcification within the tumor (**a**). The calvarium is thickened (**d**).

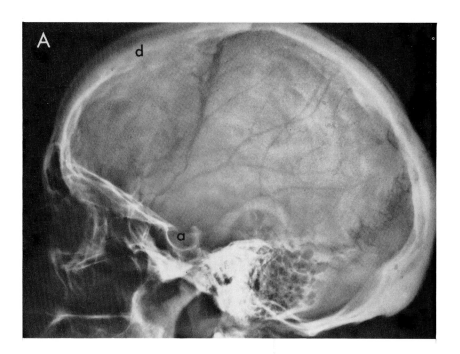

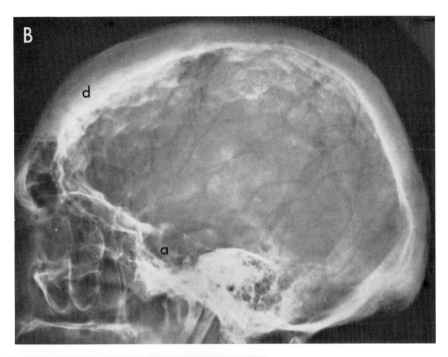

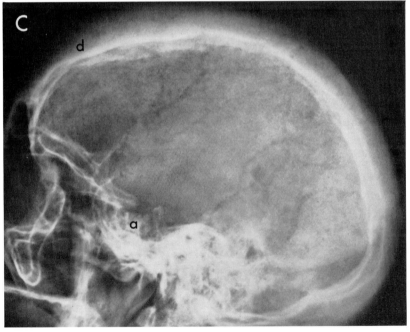

Figure 8 · Acromegaly: Skull Changes / 23

Figure 9.—Skull changes with acromeagaly.

    A, frontal view. Asymmetrical enlargement of the sella turcica with depression of the sellar floor (**arrows**) on the right side.

    B, frontal view. Excessive development of the frontal sinuses (**b**) and mastoid air cells (**e**).

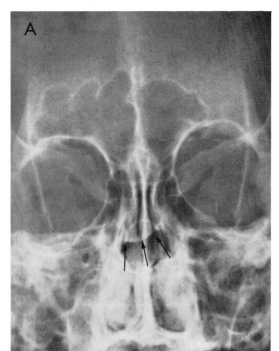

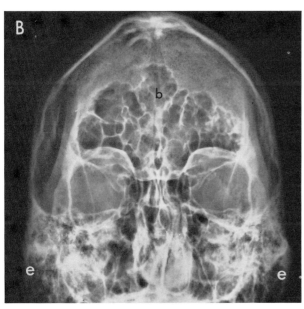

Figure 9 · Acromegaly: Skull Changes / 25

Figure 10.—Skull changes with acromegaly.

A, lateral view. In addition to enlargement of the frontal sinuses (**b**), there are an increased mandibular angle (**arrows**) and prognathism (**f**). Note the large soft tissue mass representing the hypertrophied tongue (**g**).

B, lateral view. The sella turcica is enlarged and has a double floor (**a**). Marked prognathism (**f**) and an enlarged tongue (**g**) are also apparent.

C, lateral view. The sella turcica is enlarged (**a**), and there is an increased mandibular angle. Note the spreading of the teeth.

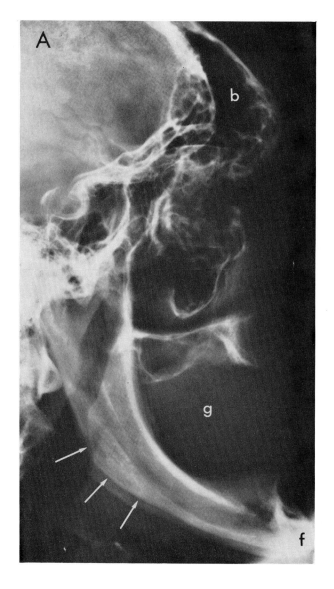

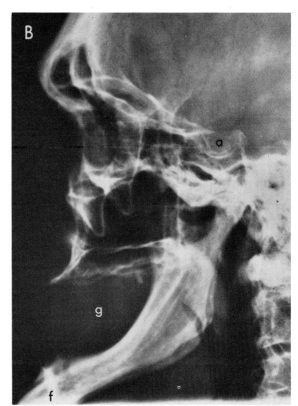

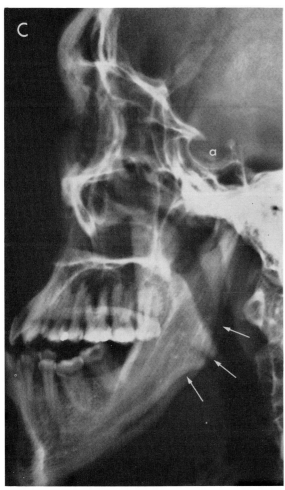

Figure 10 · Acromegaly: Skull Changes / 27

Figure 11.—Skeletal changes with acromegaly.

A, posteroanterior view of the hand. The terminal tufts of the phalanges are unusually prominent **(a)**. The joint cartilages are widened, particularly in the carpus **(b)**. The fourth metacarpal is abnormally thin **(c)**.

B, posteroanterior view of the hand. There is excessive development of the terminal tufts of the distal phalanges **(a)**. The joint cartilages are hypertrophied with apparent increase of joint space **(b)**.

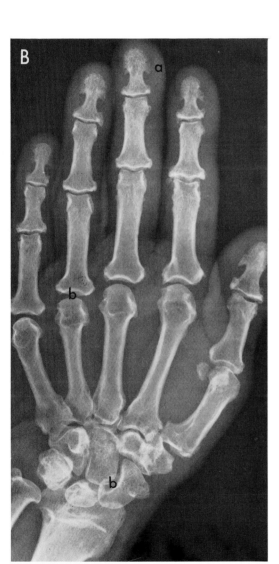

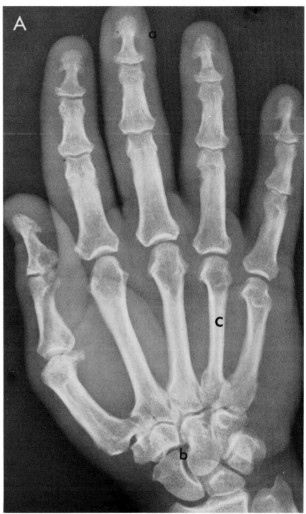

Figure 11 · Acromegaly: The Hands / 29

Figure 12.—Skeletal changes with acromegaly.

A, posteroanterior view of the foot. The joint cartilages are widened (**b**). The proximal phalanges are thinned (**c**), a manifestation of excessive bone resorption.

B, posteroanterior view of the foot. Overgrowth of the terminal tufts of the distal phalanges (**a**) and abnormally wide joint cartilage (**b**) are evident.

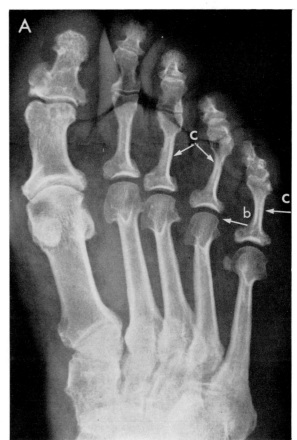

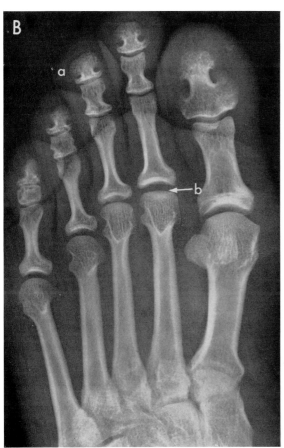

Figure 12 · Acromegaly: The Feet / 31

Figure 13.—Skeletal changes with acromegaly.

A, anteroposterior view of the pelvis. The ischium (**a**) and pubis (**b**) are narrowed bilaterally. Severe degenerative joint disease is present in both hips (**c**).

B, lateral view of the heel. The subcalcaneal soft tissue or heel pad is markedly thickened.

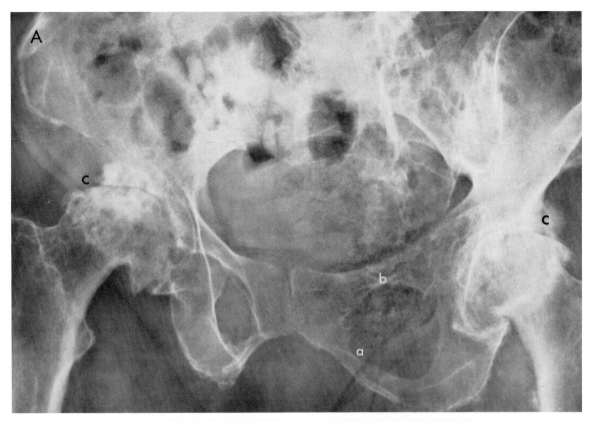

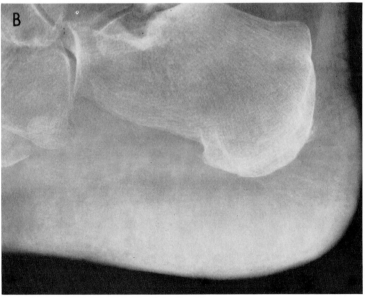

Figure 13 · Acromegaly: The Pelvis; The Heel / 33

Figure 14.—Spinal changes with acromegaly.

A, lateral view of the cervical spine. Bony overgrowth anteriorly and subsequent increase of the anteroposterior diameter of the cervical vertebral bodies has resulted in an apparent flattening of the vertebral bodies; they are, however, of normal stature (height).

B, lateral view of the thoracic spine. The posterior margins of the thoracic vertebral bodies have a scalloped appearance.

C, lateral view of the lumbar spine. The posterior margins of the lumbar vertebral bodies have a scalloped appearance.

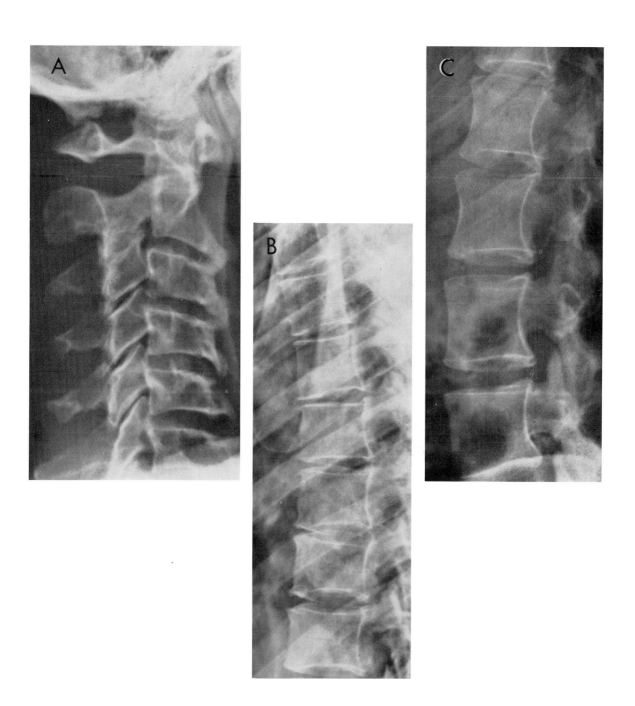

Figure 14 · Acromegaly: Spinal Changes / 35

PART 2

The Thyroid

Diseases of the Thyroid

THIS DISCUSSION concerns diseases of the thyroid gland that lead to an increase of its size.[1] The term goiter may be used to indicate a thyroid mass resulting from metabolic disease or neoplasia. The gland may be uniformly smooth or nodular and may be associated with excessive, diminution or normal production of thyroid hormone. The types of goiter may be classified as follows:

1. Simple or colloid goiter
2. Diffuse goiter with hyperthyroidism (Graves' disease)
3. Nodular goiter with hyperthyroidism, hypothyroidism or normal hormone production
4. Degenerative and inflammatory goiter
   a) Amyloid goiter
   b) Tuberculous thyroiditis
   c) Granulomatous thyroiditis (subacute or giant cell thyroiditis)
   d) Lymphocytic thyroiditis
   e) Lymphadenoid goiter (struma lymphomatosa, Hashimoto's disease)
   f) Riedel's struma
5. Neoplastic goiter
   a) Benign adenoma (trabecular, tubular, microfollicular, macrofollicular, hyperplastic)
   b) Malignant (carcinoma)
      (1) Papillary
      (2) Follicular
      (3) Solid or medullary
      (4) Hürthle cell
      (5) Giant cell and spindle cell
   c) Lymphoma (lymphosarcoma, reticulum cell sarcoma, Hodgkin's disease)
   d) Tumors metastatic to the thyroid
6. Thyroid acropachy

SIMPLE OR COLLOID GOITER

These goiters develop commonly in geographic regions where iodine content of water and soil is low and calcium carbonate content of water is high. A diffuse enlargement frequently appears at puberty in both sexes, but

---

[1] Anderson, W. A. D.: *Pathology* (5th ed.; St. Louis: C. V. Mosby Company, 1966). Lindsay, S.: *Carcinoma of the Thyroid Gland* (Springfield, Ill.: Charles C Thomas, Publisher, 1960). Netter, F. H.: Endocrine System and Selected Metabolic Diseases, in *Ciba Collection of Medical Illustrations* (Summit, N. J.: Ciba Pharmaceutical Products, Inc., 1965), Vol. 4.

two or three times more often in males. The goiters of females may become large, particularly in association with multiple pregnancies. Later, the goiters become nodular and may be symmetrical or asymmetrical. A nodular portion arising from the lower part of the goiter may descend beneath the sternum into the anterior mediastinum. Occasionally it will extend into the middle or posterior mediastinum. The displacement into the mediastinum may occur suddenly, and in some instances, the entire mass is displaced even though a mass in the neck is not evident. The patient may complain of dysphagia or difficulty in breathing.

PATHOLOGIC CHANGES.—The diffuse colloid goiter may be three or more times the size of a normal thyroid gland. Diffuse hyperplasia is present which, in time, may become multinodular. In long-standing disease, hemorrhage, cyst formation, fibrosis and calcification occur. Histologic examination reveals many types of benign adenomas, from a highly undifferentiated trabecular pattern to that of a hyperplastic adenoma. Rarely, malignant growths may be present within a nodule (Fig. 21, C).

The goiter is caused by excess stimulation by pituitary thyroid-stimulating hormone resulting from a deficiency of thyroid hormone secretion. The impairment of thyroid synthesis may be the result of congenitally defective enzyme systems, iodine deficiency in diet, drugs, or goitrogenic substances in the diet.

DIFFUSE GOITER WITH HYPERTHYROIDISM (GRAVES' DISEASE)

This syndrome is characterized by hyperthyroidism and exophthalmos and is about eight times as common in females as in males. In endemic goitrous areas, the sex ratio is less. The syndrome may appear at any age, but most often occurs in young adults. Evidence exists that the syndrome is on a genetic basis with a recessive factor.

CLINICAL FINDINGS.—Common symptoms and signs include exophthalmos, goiter, a fine tremor, nervousness, emotional instability, sweating, heat intolerance, palpitations and hyperkinesis. Loss of weight and strength, anorexia, nausea, vomiting, symptoms from cardiac failure and menstrual disturbances may occur. In addition to exophthalmos, there may be widened palpebral fissures, blinking, lid lag, failure of convergence and failure to wrinkle the brow on upward gaze. Cardiovascular changes include a widely spaced pulse beat, sinus tachycardia, atrial arrhythmias, systolic murmurs, increased intensity of apical first sounds, cardiac enlargement and heart failure. The thymus and lymph nodes are often large.

The basal metabolic rate is increased, and the serum protein-bound iodine and butanol-extractable iodine levels are high. There is increased red cell or resin uptake of radioactive triiodothyronine and rapid, increased thyroid uptake of radioiodine.

In some patients with hyperthyroidism or in whom it has been treated, localized myxedema develops. This myxedema consists of a circumscribed deposition of mucinous material in the deeper layers of the skin over the lower portion of the legs or dorsum of the feet. Usually, exophthalmos and clubbed fingers are present in these patients.

Hypercalciuria and hyperphosphaturia are present in some patients, and in these, the serum calcium, phosphorus and alkaline phosphatase levels are usually normal. Others may have hypercalcemia and an elevated alkaline phosphatase content. Bone lesions may appear as osteoporosis, osteomalacia or osteitis fibrosa on histologic sections, but on roentgenograms the bones usually appear to be normal. When the disease develops in childhood, the bone age is usually within normal range but may be accelerated.

PATHOLOGIC CHANGES.—The gland is usually enlarged two to four times its normal size. The enlargement is highly vascular and is usually symmetrical, but one lobe may be disproportionately large. Histologic examination reveals diffuse hyperplasia with a decreased amount of epithelial cells of the columnar and colloid follicles. Intrafollicular papillary proliferation is often present. Lymphocytic infiltration is seen with lymph follicle formation.

NODULAR GOITER (ADENOMATOUS GOITER)

This type of goiter may be associated with an excessive, a normal or a deficient production of thyroid hormone. The nodularity results from recurrent episodes of hyperplasia and hypertrophy affecting the gland irregularly. There may be a single adenoma or multiple adenomas containing a variety of adenomas whose function varies.

CLINICAL FINDINGS.—These patients are usually past 40 years of age and often come from a region where goiters are endemic. In the patients with functioning nodules, some features of Graves' disease may be seen. Characteristically, exophthalmos and clubbing of the fingers and toes are not present. Muscular weakness and weight loss are less and, in general, metabolic abnormalities are fewer than in Graves' disease. The thymus and lymph nodes are not enlarged. The total uptake of radioactive iodine is less and is usually concentrated primarily in the hyperfunctioning adenoma.

The disease usually occurs in previously nontoxic nodular goiters.

PATHOLOGIC CHANGES.—Clinical distinction from a true neoplastic adenoma is impossible. The gross and histologic appearances vary. The enlargement may be pronounced and irregular. Areas of degeneration, hemorrhage, cyst formation, hyalinization and calcification are common. Hyperplasia may

Diseases of the Thyroid Gland / 41

be seen in some areas, and other areas may contain colloid. Some adenomas may be highly undifferentiated and rarely malignant, whereas others are well differentiated and functional.

DEGENERATIVE AND INFLAMMATORY GOITERS

The thyroid is resistant to most infections, but abscess, gummas, tuberculosis and various infections can occur.

STRUMA LYMPHOMATOSA (Hashimoto's disease).—Struma lymphomatosa develops mostly in women, usually after age 40. Most commonly, mild hypothyroidism and pressure symptoms referable to the trachea are present. The thyroid is enlarged, sometimes to several times its normal size. It is slightly nodular but usually uniformly enlarged.

Serum flocculation tests and protein patterns may be abnormal. The disease shows evidence of autoimmune phenomena. In about 75% of patients, laboratory studies show both precipitating (thyroglobulin) and complement fixation antibodies and in about 10% only complement fixation antibodies.

Pathologic changes.—The thyroid is uniformly enlarged and the capsule intact. Histologically, lymphoid tissue is infiltrated extensively, follicles are atrophic, and colloid is diminished. Connective tissue may be increased.

RIEDEL'S STRUMA.—This is a rare cause of thyroidal enlargement that is predominant in males. The average age of the patient is somewhat lower than with struma lymphomatosa. Riedel's struma is the result of a chronic fibrosing process of the thyroid which may compress or displace the trachea and esophagus.

The thyroid is hard and adherent to adjacent tissues but not to skin. The patients complain of pressure, but hypothyroidism, if present, is mild.

Pathologic changes.—Only a part of the thyroid gland may be abnormal. The affected part is hard, dense and sclerotic. Histologically, distinct fibrosis is noted. The thyroid parenchyma is replaced to a variable extent, but small follicles often persist.

NEOPLASTIC GOITER

BENIGN ADENOMA.—This is a true tumor surrounded by a fibrous capsule. It may occur at any age—most frequently at 40–50—but is rare in children. About 65% of adenomas are in women. The tumor is usually single, but may be multiple and range in size from 1 to 10 cm or more.

Although the small adenomas may not cause symptoms, the larger ones may press on the trachea or esophagus. Some well-differentiated functional adenomas may produce enough hormone to cause symptoms of thyrotoxicosis. Adenomas may be ectopic and situated along the thyroglossal tract from the base of the tongue to the diaphragm. Lingual goiters, thyroglossal duct cysts (Fig. 20), pyramidal lobe adenomas, esophageal and tracheal rests and ectopic thyroid tissue in ovaries have been described.

Pathologic changes.—Adenomas may be divided into different types, depending on the degree of histologic differentiation. In order of increasing differentiation, they have been called trabecular, tubular, microfollicular, macrofollicular and hyperplastic. The trabecular and tubular adenomas are nonfunctional, and no uptake of radioactive iodine is detected. Malignant propensities are noted in some of these. Some microfollicular adenomas are functional and absorb radioactive iodine, but less than does normal thyroid tissue. Macrofollicular or colloid adenomas are the most frequent benign thyroid tumors. They differ from diffuse colloid goiters only in that they are encapsulated. Function and radioactive uptake vary. Cancer does not arise in follicular adenoma, and psammoma bodies are never found in these tumors.

MALIGNANT TUMORS (carcinoma).—About 14% of single nodules and 4% of multinodular goiters contain carcinoma (Fig. 21, *C*). Malignancy develops in fewer than 2% of toxic goiters.

1. *Papillary carcinoma* is the most common form, comprising 50–60% of malignant thyroid tumors. It is present at all ages, but it occurs at an earlier age than other thyroid growths and is usually seen in young adults. It is more common in females than in males. The tumors are often very small and may be detected by metastatic spread to neighboring lymph nodes. Multiple foci are often present. The papillary form is the least aggressive of thyroid malignancy. Metastasis to the cervical and upper mediastinal nodes (Fig. 22) can occur early and then metastasize to the lung. Function and uptake of radioactive iodine by the primary and metastatic tumors are minimal. Blood-borne metastasis to the skeleton and brain, or other sites, is unusual.

The *histologic examination* reveals papillary cords with vascular connective tissue that is lined by from one to many layers of cuboidal and columnar cells. Usually, colloid is not present, but in some tumors, areas of follicular carcinoma contain well-differentiated follicles. Spherical concentric calcifications, called psammoma bodies, are present in about 60% of this type of carcinoma. They are usually in the tumor but may be in the adjacent normal gland.

2. *Follicular carcinoma* is the second most common type of thyroid neoplasm, making up 15–20% of all malignant tumors of the thyroid gland. It, too, appears most often in females, usually in those between 20 and 40 years old. As in papillary carcinoma, multiple foci may be in the thyroid. These may metastasize to cervical and mediastinal lymph nodes and then to

Diseases of the Thyroid Gland / 43

the lungs. The follicular type of tumor is often larger than the papillary and metastasizes to bone more often than does any other thyroid tumor (Figs. 27–29). Uptake of radioactive iodine, some in therapeutic amounts, is demonstrable in most of the tumors.

Follicular carcinoma is relatively nonaggressive, but is more aggressive than papillary carcinoma. On *histologic examination,* the size of the follicles varies considerably, but their shape is usually irregular. The cells of the follicular lining are larger than normal and contain large nuclei. Mitoses are uncommon. Psammoma bodies are less common than in papillary carcinoma yet more common than in other malignant neoplasms. They are present in about 25% of follicular carcinomas.

3. *Solid adenocarcinoma* constitutes about 15% of malignant thyroid tumors. It occurs in patients usually past 40 and most often in females. The tumors are usually large, single and limited to one lobe. Metastasis is usually blood-borne, most commonly to the lung and skeleton but also to the liver and kidney as well as to other organs. The pulmonary lesions consist of one nodule or a few discrete nodules, and the skeletal metastatic lesion is multiple or single. Function in these lesions is minimal or absent.

Histologic examination reveals a solid trabecular pattern of closely packed cells with variation in the size of nuclei and with hyperchromatism. Some areas may contain a follicular structure. Solid adenocarcinoma is more malignant than the papillary, follicular or Hürthle cell type of cancer.

Another distinct form of solid adenocarcinoma, called *medullary carcinoma,* has become important in the past decade. It is slow-growing, is only moderately malignant, may be multicentric and is characterized by amyloid stroma limited to the tumor or its metastasis. Medullary carcinoma metastasizes frequently to the regional lymph nodes. It is sometimes associated with pheochromocytomas, which may be multiple. Other associated conditions may be mucosal neuromas, parathyroid hyperplasia or adenoma, Cushing's syndrome, carcinoid syndrome and, less frequently, neurofibromatosis. The tumor secretes calcitonin, which may induce hypocalcemia. It is recorded in familial aggregates, and an autosomal dominant inheritance has been postulated.

4. *Hürthle cell carcinoma* constitutes about 10% of thyroid carcinomas. It is four to eight times as common in females as in males and is most prevalent between 25 and 50 years. Usually, only a single nodule is present, which may be small or large. The tumor is usually of low grade malignancy but may metastasize through the vascular system to the skeleton and, less often, to the lungs. Occasionally the tumor extends to regional lymph nodes. As indicated by radioactive iodine uptake, function of the tumor is low or absent.

The *histologic examination* reveals cuboidal or columnar cells in a trabecular pattern, with columns separated by rich capillary blood supply or stratified in plexiform groups separated by capillaries. Many pathologists do not regard this appearance as a separate type of carcinoma. They prefer rather to classify it as a subordinate type of follicular, papillary or anaplastic carcinoma, depending on whether any of these other forms are present, which is frequently the case.

5. *Giant cell* and *spindle cell carcinomas* are extremely anaplastic and rapidly fatal tumors. They constitute fewer than 10% of thyroid carcinomas and occur after age 50 in most patients. They are rapidly growing, nonfunctional tumors that involve the trachea, esophagus, hypopharynx and surrounding tissues. Distant metastasis is uncommon, and death usually occurs within 1 year of the diagnosis.

LYMPHOMA.—Lymphosarcoma (Fig. 18), reticulum cell sarcoma and Hodgkin's disease may be present in the thyroid gland when the disease is generalized but rarely as primary tumors. The lesions are identical to respective lesions appearing elsewhere.

THYROID ACROPACHY

This interesting disease may occur in thyrotoxic patients. The disease may rarely be present before treatment, but usually appears later. The patients have exophthalmos, pretibial myxedema, swelling of soft tissues and clubbing of the fingers or toes. Periosteal new bone, which is irregular and spiculated, involves most often the first and fifth metacarpals, but also other metacarpals and phalanges (Fig. 31). Soft tissue swelling may often be seen overlying the periosteal reaction (Fig. 32). It may occur in the feet and tibia and fibula, as well as in other bones. The heel pads of the feet may be very thick.

ROENTGEN CHANGES WITH THYROID DISEASE

THE NECK MASS[2]

GRAVES' DISEASE.—In Graves' disease, the thyroid is usually diffusely enlarged and does not displace the trachea or esophagus laterally. In many

---

[2] Kreel, L.: Radiological investigation of thyroid enlargement, Australasian Radiol. 10:107, May, 1966. Schein, C., *et al.*: Relation of thyroid enlargement to tracheal configuration: Anatomico-roentgenologic correlation, New England J. Med. 255:1072, Dec. 6, 1956. Schinz, H. R., *et al.*: *Roentgen-Diagnostics* (New York: Grune & Stratton, Inc., 1953), Vol. 3, pp. 2087–91 and 2736–40; Vol. 4, pp. 3177–78.

instances, however, the enlarged lateral lobes impinge on the upper esophagus bilaterally, producing a smooth, symmetrical narrowing. On lateral roentgenograms, a soft tissue mass may be seen anterior to the trachea. Occasionally, the enlarged thyroid may encroach on the anterior aspect of the esophagus, increasing the space between esophagus and trachea. Slight narrowing may be noted in the trachea. The changes are most obvious in thyrotoxic patients receiving medical treatment, but also in some with Hashimoto's thyroiditis. The degree of narrowing is not proportional to the size of the thyroid gland or degree of symptoms.

Of considerable interest as a late manifestation of hyperthyroidism is acropachy. Acropachy, a rare finding in patients with old or recurring hyperthyroidism, occurs more often in men than in women despite the fact that Graves' disease is four to five times more common in women. Acropachy is manifested by a swelling of the extremities, clubbing of the fingers or toes or both, the swelling being associated with periosteal new bone formation. This type of abnormally spiculated periosteal new bone formation more often affects the hands than the feet, and in the hands most frequently involves the metacarpal bones, though the phalanges often reveal similar periostitis.

Radiologically the periosteal new bone formation in acropachy is characterized by a somewhat spiculated appearance (Figs. 31 and 32). It differs from hypertrophic pulmonary osteoarthropathy in which the periosteal new bone is more uniform and smooth than the shaggy new bone observed in acropachy. Also, the former less commonly is confined to the hands and feet, often affecting primarily the forearms and lower limbs.

NODULAR THYROIDS.—The largest goiters are usually slow-growing, asymmetrical and nontoxic. Esophageal constriction is minimal. The trachea and esophagus are displaced laterally to the same degree (Fig. 15), and the thyroid cartilage may also be displaced, but to a lesser extent. The displacement to the right is usually greater than to the left, possibly because of the aortic arch on the left side. The mass may extend between the trachea and esophagus or behind the esophagus, producing anterior or posterior displacement (Fig. 15).

MALIGNANT TUMORS.—Most malignant lesions are well localized or encapsulated and produce displacement similar to that seen with adenomas. More aggressive lesions, such as giant cell and spindle cell tumors, small cell carcinomas and lymphosarcoma, may infiltrate the trachea and esophagus. The infiltration of the trachea may be seen on plain roentgenograms as an irregular mass encroaching on the air space (Fig. 17). On barium examination of the esophagus, the trachea may appear to be constricted and its mucosa destroyed (Fig. 16). The trachea and esophagus will become fixed (Fig. 17) and, along with the tumor, will not move up or down on swallowing or coughing. The trachea may not distend or collapse with the Valsalva or Müller maneuver. The trachea may also become fixed with Riedel's thyroiditis.

MEDIASTINAL GOITER.—This type of goiter is the most common mediastinal tumor. It is usually an extension from the lower pole of a nodular cervical goiter. A mass is present in the neck, and on roentgenograms or on fluoroscopy the extension into the mediastinum may be seen in the midline (Fig. 19). Sometimes the goiter will disappear from the neck and appear as an isolated mediastinal mass. Its usual position is in the anterior mediastinum, but may be between the trachea and esophagus or behind the esophagus. The upper mediastinum is widened by a central shadow whose lateral margins are convex and sharp. The trachea is displaced laterally by the excentric mass as are the adjacent tissues, accounting for the central position of the soft tissue shadow. The trachea and esophagus are often constricted. Fluoroscopic examination should reveal a substernal thyroid that moves with coughing and swallowing. Rarely, isolated aberrant thyroid masses are present in the mediastinum. These are not attached to the cervical thyroid and do not move with the gland.

Occasionally, a single adenoma may be found in the anterior mediastinum that has no connection with the organ in the neck. This suggests development from an ectopic thyroid anlage. The gross and microscopic appearance as a rule is that of a nodular colloid goiter.

LINGUAL THYROIDS.—These develop along the course of the thyroglossal duct. They may be seen on lateral roentgenograms as a mass at the root of the tongue. Depending on their position, they may displace the hyoid bone upward or downward.

CALCIFICATION

Calcification is common in benign and malignant goiters.[3] The calcification may be dense, amorphous, sharply defined plaques, generally in or around benign nodules in fibrotic areas (Fig. 19). This type of calcification is present often in the benign and malignant lesions. Other distinctive calcifications, the psammoma bodies, are seen almost exclusively in thyroid glands containing primary malignant tumors (Fig. 20 and 21). These are numerous, small, not densely calcified deposits of approximately equal size and usually grouped in streaks or whorls. In some instances, the psammoma bodies are in adjacent nonmalignant areas of the gland. Although the psam-

---

[3] Holtz, S., and Powers, W. E.: Calcification in papillary carcinoma of thyroid, Am. J. Roentgenol. 80:997, December, 1958. Margolin, F. R., *et al.*: Patterns of thyroid calcification, Invest. Radiol. 2:208, May-June, 1967; Soft tissue roentgenography of thyroid nodules, Am. J. Roentgenol. 102:844, April, 1968.

moma bodies are often noted in histologic examination, on roentgenograms they may be seen in only about 20% of thyroid tumors.

The differential diagnosis between thyroid cancer and goiter in the presence of a nodular thyroid gland may challenge the skill of the clinician, particularly in endemic goiter areas. In such regions, a high percentage of the population may have thyroid tumors that are not operated on. For this reason, one would hope that the calcifications oft seen in enlarged thyroids might give a clue as to whether or not the lesion is benign in much the same manner that fine calcifications reveal breast malignancies with a high degree of accuracy.

ARTERIOGRAPHY

Arteriography may be useful in identifying malignant tumors or metastasis. Gas injected into the soft tissue adjacent to the thyroid gland may indicate the size and shape of the mass.[4]

METASTATIC LESIONS

Local invasion of the trachea and esophagus may be diagnosed on plain roentgenograms or on barium examination of the esophagus. Regional and mediastinal lymph nodes may be demonstrated by arteriography (Fig. 22).

PULMONARY METASTASIS.—This may be of two types. Papillary and follicular carcinomas often metastasize in a characteristic manner that is not duplicated by other neoplasms (Figs. 23–26). Initially, the lesions may appear as small, indistinct, miliary shadows in the lower lung fields. These lesions may remain stationary for many years or they may enlarge slowly, forming nodular lesions that may persist unchanged while others are growing. Some nodular lesions may grow to form conglomerate lesions. Miliary lesions are produced by the low-grade malignant growth, such as papillary adenocarcinoma and, to a lesser extent, follicular adenocarcinoma.

The more malignant adenocarcinomas of the thyroid gland produce metastatic tumors to the lung indistinguishable from those arising in other organs. The metastatic deposits are discrete solitary or multiple lesions that may grow rapidly.

SKELETAL METASTASIS.[5]—Metastasis to bones is slightly less frequent than pulmonary metastasis. Bone lesions may occur many years after the

---

[4] Djindjian, R., et al.: L'artériographie du corps thyroide: Ses applications diagnostiques, Ann. radiol. 7:693, Sept.-Oct., 1964. Rozenshtraukh, L. S., and Ponomarev, L. E.: Pneumothyroidography in diseases of thyroid gland, Fed. Proc. 23(supp.):2393, Mar.-Apr., 1964.

[5] Sherman, R. S., and Ivker, M.: Roentgen appearance of thyroid metastases in bone, Am. J. Roentgenol. 63:196, February, 1950.

onset of cancer. Undifferentiated carcinomas are more likely to metastasize to bone, but they constitute only a small percentage of thyroid carcinomas. Most metastatic bone tumors are papillary or follicular. Although follicular adenocarcinoma is much less common than papillary adenocarcinoma, its propensity to metastasize to bone is greater. The most common sites are the spine, ribs, sternum, skull, pelvis, femur and humerus (Figs. 27–30). In many of these patients, pulmonary lesions are not evident, and possibly the axial neoplastic spread is through the paravertebral venous plexus. The lesions of bone are usually of medullary origin, with medullary and cortical destruction but no periosteal reaction. They are almost always of oval shape, small to medium in size, and extend somewhat beyond the bone. The lesions are osteolytic with occasional faint septa, calcific flecks or small dense areas at the borders, which are indistinct. An unusual feature is the ability of the metastatic growths to cross a joint and involve adjacent bones. This involvement may take place between the ribs and spine or between the pelvis and hip, the ilium and sacrum, or between other regions. The lesions are highly vascular.

Figure 15.—Nodular goiter.

A, anteroposterior roentgenogram of the neck and upper mediastinum after barium ingestion. A large nodular goiter in the right side of the neck displaces the esophagus (**a**) and trachea (**b**) to the left. The trachea and esophagus are almost equally displaced, and the trachea is not significantly narrowed on this view. Nodular goiters tend to displace rather than compress the esophagus and trachea. Part of the goiter has descended below the clavicles and produced a symmetrical widening of the mediastinum (**c**).

B (same patient as in *A*), lateral roentgenogram after barium ingestion. The goiter has extended between the esophagus and trachea. The esophagus is displaced posteriorly (**a**). The trachea is displaced anteriorly and is slightly compressed, particularly at the level of the thoracic inlet, where forward displacement is limited by the sternum (**b**). In other patients, the mass may be in front of the trachea or behind the esophagus.

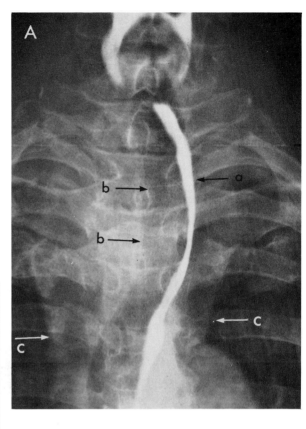

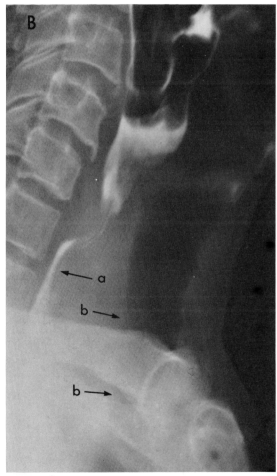

Figure 15 · Nodular Goiter / 51

Figure 16.—Follicular carcinoma of the thyroid (all figures from same patient).

A, anteroposterior roentgenogram after barium ingestion. The lower part of the pharynx and the esophagus are compressed by the neoplasm in the right side of the neck (**arrows**).

B, lateral roentgenogram, showing the tumor extending between the esophagus and trachea as well as anterior to the trachea. The tracheal lumen is narrowed (**arrows**).

C, tomogram of the trachea, anteroposterior projection. The trachea is narrowed; in addition, some tumor tissue has invaded the wall and is surrounded by air in the lumen (**arrows**).

D, lateral roentgenogram, lightly exposed. The calcified tracheal cartilages are visible anteriorly (**a**). The tracheal lumen (the dark shadow) is displaced posteriorly by neoplasm infiltrating the tracheal wall (**b**).

E, anteroposterior roentgenogram after the tracheal mucosa was opacified with opaque contrast material. The neoplastic tissue invading the right side of the trachea seen on the tomogram (*C*) is better demonstrated here (**arrows**).

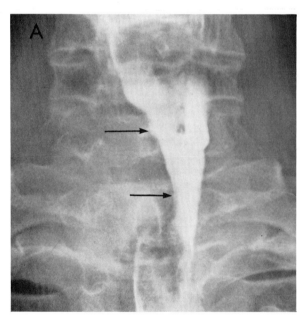
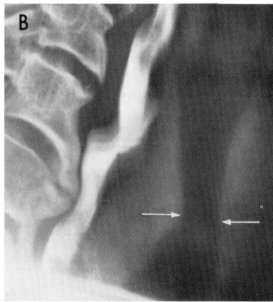

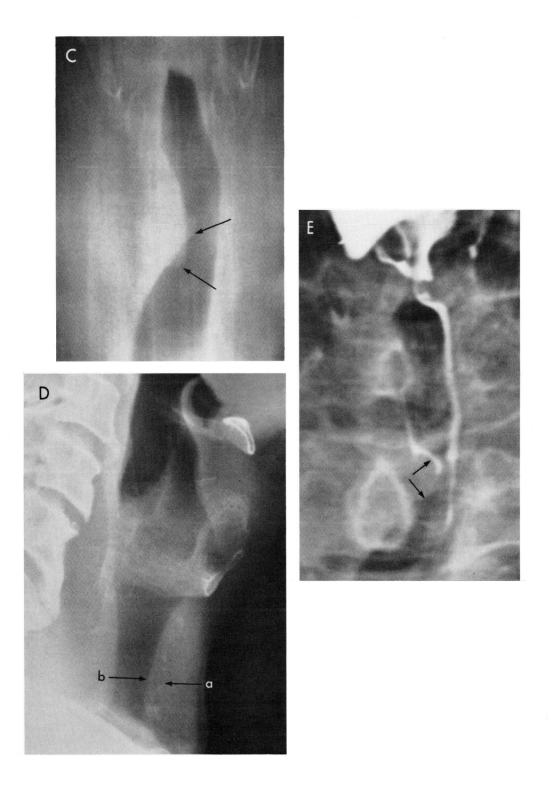

Figure 16 · Follicular Carcinoma / 53

Figure 17.—Medullary carcinoma of the thyroid: Sarcomatous degeneration of an adenomatous goiter.

A, medullary carcinoma of the thyroid gland. Anteroposterior roentgenogram of the neck and upper mediastinum. A sharply demarcated mass encroaches on the air space of the trachea from its left border, but causes minimal displacement. The outer border of the mass is visible in the upper mediastinum surrounded by lung (**arrows**). The malignant tumor has invaded and "fixed" the trachea, which explains the marked narrowing of the lumen with minimal displacement.

B, sarcomatous degeneration of an adenomatous goiter. Posteroanterior roentgenogram. A huge redundant mass arises in the neck and extends over the clavicle and right anterior chest. It is not in the thorax. At least two spherical, sharply demarcated metastatic lesions, characteristic of metastatic sarcoma, are present in the lungs (**arrows**).

This 90-year-old woman had had goiter for 70 years. The sarcoma had appeared recently.

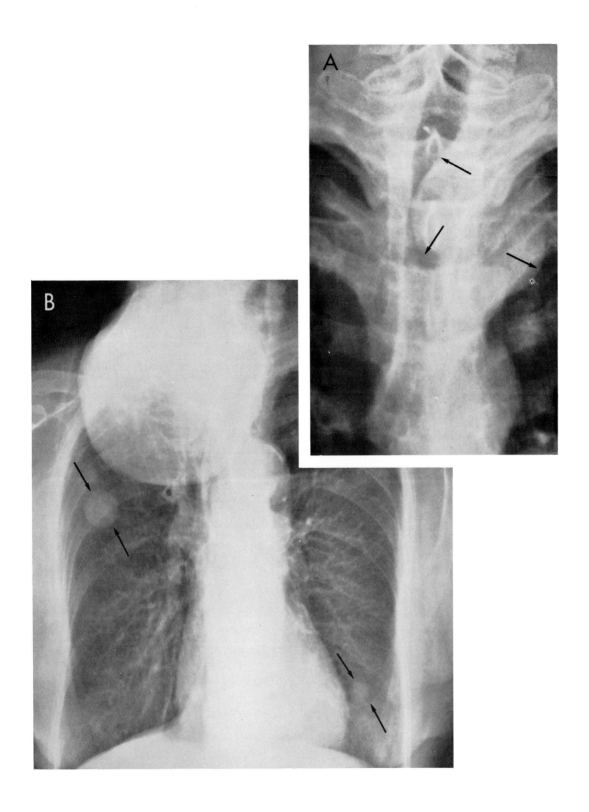

Figure 17 · Carcinoma: Sarcoma in Goiter / 55

Figure 18.—Primary lymphosarcoma of the thyroid gland (all figures from same patient).

A, anteroposterior roentgenogram of the neck after barium ingestion. There is no significant displacement of the pharynx, esophagus or trachea. The neoplasm may be exerting some extrinsic pressure on the right border of the upper esophagus.

B, lateral roentgenogram obtained at the same examination. A soft tissue mass is visible anterior to the upper trachea and thyroid cartilage (**a**). The tracheal rings are calcified and are immediately adjacent to the air space anteriorly (**b**). The barium-filled esophagus is in its normal position immediately behind the trachea.

C, anteroposterior roentgenogram obtained 5 months after *A*. The esophagus and trachea are displaced considerably to the left.

D, lateral roentgenogram obtained 5 months after *B*. The tumor has grown considerably, increasing the distance between the esophagus and trachea (**a**). The tracheal air space is diminished by neoplastic infiltration of the trachea. The tracheal lumen is no longer adjacent to the calcified cartilage rings because of tumor infiltration of the wall (**b**). A benign tumor may compress the trachea, including the tracheal cartilages, but would not infiltrate and thicken its wall.

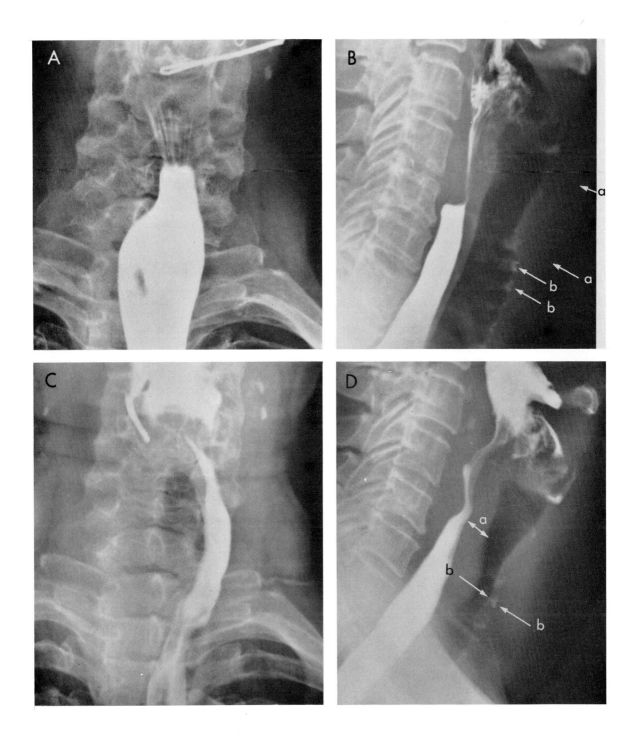

Figure 18 · Primary Lymphosarcoma / 57

Figure 19.—Intrathoracic nodular goiter.

A, nodular goiter with substernal extension. Posteroanterior roentgenogram, showing a large, sharply circumscribed soft tissue mass in the neck and upper mediastinum (**arrows**). Tracheal displacement to the left (**a**) is limited by the aorta (**b**).

B, nodular goiter with anterior intrathoracic extension. Posteroanterior roentgenogram of the chest, demonstrating displacement of the esophagus and trachea to the right in the neck (**arrow**). The mass has extended in the anterior mediastinum to the hilar level (**a**). The upper mediastinum is almost symmetrically widened (**b**), but farther down it extends more to the right.

C (same patient as in *B*), lateral roentgenogram, showing the soft tissue mass in the anterior mediastinum (**arrow**). The goiter has also extended into the middle mediastinum, separating the esophagus and trachea (**c**). Dense, irregular, amorphous plaques of calcification and semicircular calcifications are visible in the anterior portion of the goiter (**d**). This type of calcification is usually in or around benign nodules in fibrotic areas.

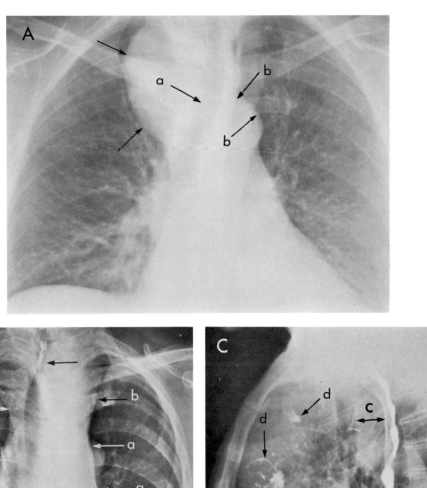

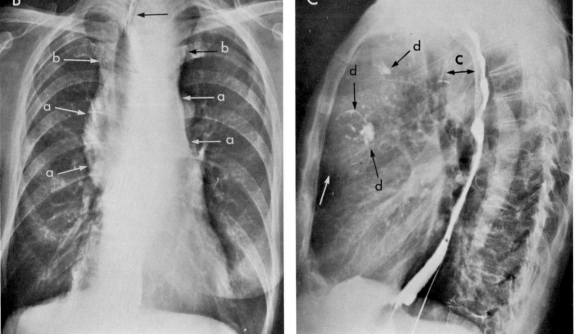

Figure 19 · Intrathoracic Nodular Goiter / 59

Figure 20.—Thyroglossal duct cyst; Papillary carcinoma in a thyroglossal duct cyst.

A, lateral roentgenogram of a thyroglossal duct cyst filled with opaque contrast medium. The cyst is derived from remnants of the thyroglossal duct and is situated in the midline. The persistent channels of the thyroglossal duct do not penetrate the skin except when the skin is ruptured by pressure necrosis from an expanding cyst or ulceration secondary to infection.

The human thyroid gland originates from invagination of the pharyngeal epithelium, with some contribution from the lateral pharyngeal pouches. Progressive descent of the midline thyroid anlage gives rise to the thyroglossal duct, which extends from the foramen caecum at the base of the tongue to the isthmus of the thyroid. Remnants of tissue may persist along the course of this tract as lingual thyroid, as thyroglossal cysts and nodules or as a structure contiguous with the thyroid isthmus called the pyramidal lobe.

B, lateral roentgenogram of the neck of a patient with a palpable midline mass beneath the mandible. A soft tissue mass is visible adjacent to the base of the tongue and in front of the hyoid bone. Within the mass are several small calcific densities with characteristics of psammoma bodies, indicating a malignant thyroid neoplasm (**arrows**). A circular linear calcification is superimposed on the trachea and is probably around a benign nodule (**a**).

C, a detailed view of the mass in *B*. The psammoma bodies are numerous, small, faintly calcified bodies of almost equal size (**arrows**). They are found almost exclusively in primary malignant tumors of adjacent thyroid tissue.

A papillary carcinoma arising in a thyroglossal duct cyst was found.

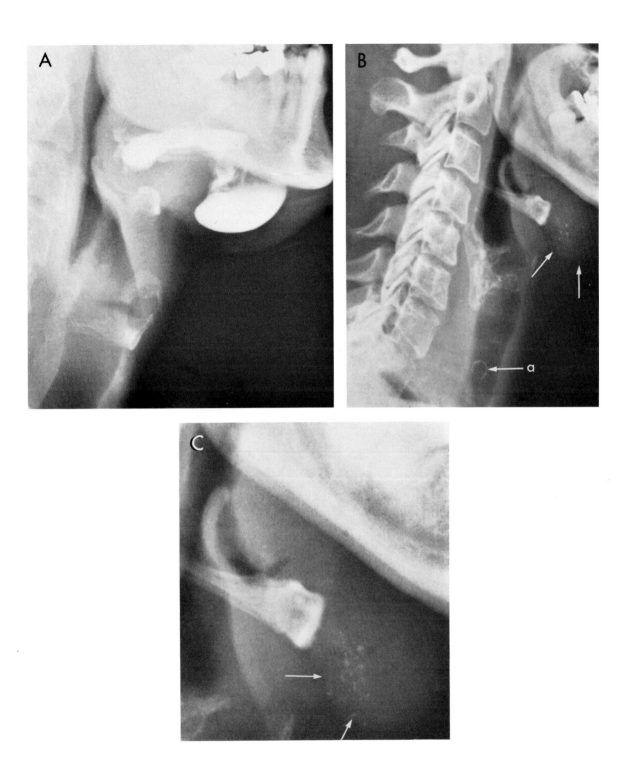

Figure 20 · Thyroglossal Duct Cysts / 61

Figure 21.—Calcification in malignant thyroid tumors.

A, papillary carcinoma of the thyroid. Anteroposterior roentgenogram of the neck, demonstrating numerous unusually dense and large psammoma bodies in a large tumor to the right of the trachea (**arrows**) and higher to the left of the trachea at the level of the thyroid cartilage. The psammoma bodies indicate the malignant nature of the neoplasm.

B (same patient as in *A*), lateral roentgenogram, showing the psammoma bodies superimposed upon and behind the trachea. The neoplasm has invaded and partially destroyed the body and posterior processes of the fifth cervical vertebra, which collapsed. Psammoma bodies are visible within the vertebral body (**arrows**).

C, papillary carcinoma arising within a benign calcified adenoma. Anteroposterior roentgenogram of the neck, demonstrating a mass to the right of the trachea, displacing it slightly to the left. Within the mass is a spherical, amorphous, dense, sharply defined plaque-like calcification of the type seen around benign adenomas (**arrow**).

This was a benign adenoma, but within it was an adenocarcinoma, possibly arising as a result of malignant degeneration. Psammoma bodies almost always indicate that a malignant lesion is present, but often benign types of calcific densities are also present. Calcification around benign nodules does not exclude a malignant growth in other parts of the thyroid.

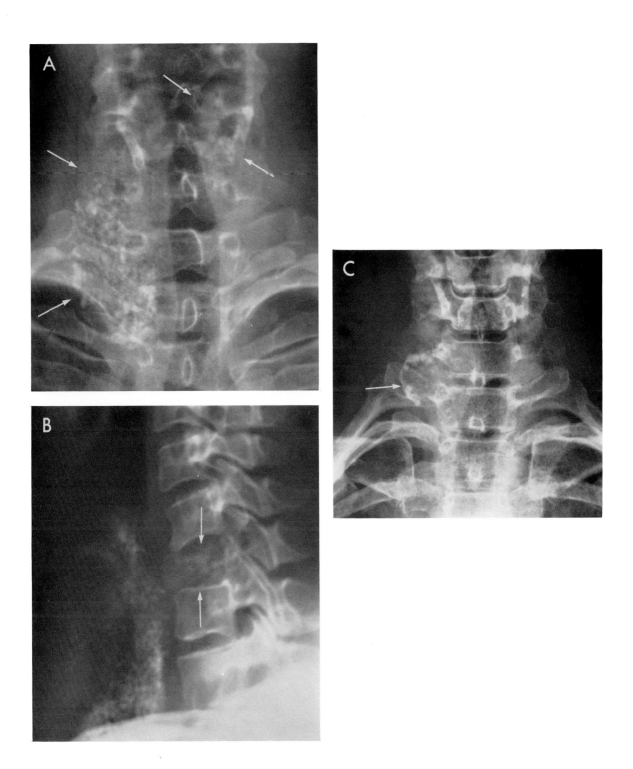

Figure 21 · Carcinoma: Calcification / 63

Figure 22.—Metastasis of thyroid papillary adenocarcinoma to left cervical lymph nodes (all figures from same patient).

A, anteroposterior view of a selective angiogram. The catheter is in the external carotid artery (**arrow**). Branches of the external carotid artery supply numerous small vessels supplying the metastatic neoplasm (**a**). Only the upper part of the neoplasm derives its blood supply from this source.

B, the catheter has been inserted into the ascending thyroid artery (**b**) and contrast medium injected. This is an early roentgenogram of a series and shows the ascending thyroid artery (**c**) and branches (**d**), some of which are tortuous, supplying the neoplasm.

C, a later roentgenogram, obtained after many of the arteries have emptied. The metastatic neoplasm is now diffusely opaque because of pooling of the opaque contrast material in the numerous arterioles, capillaries and venules (**e**).

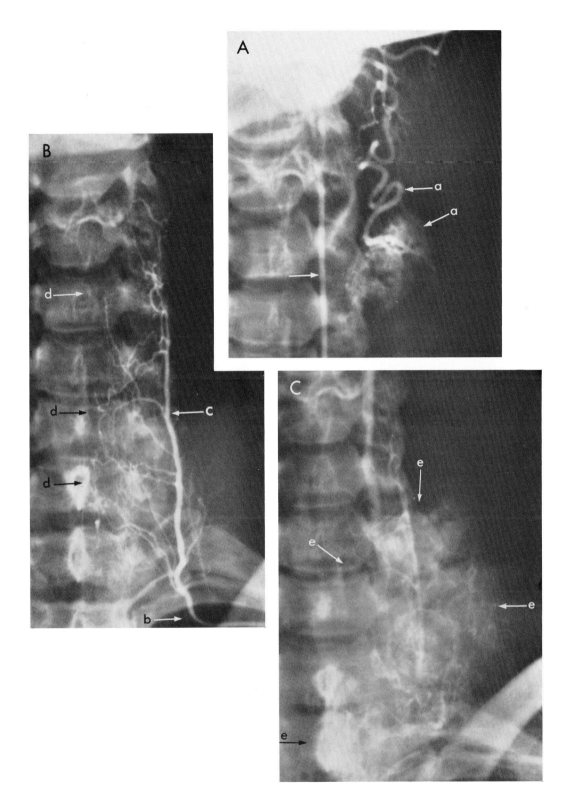

Figure 22 · Carcinoma: Lymph Node Metastases / 65

Figure 23.—Metastasis to the lung from thyroid papillary adenocarcinoma.

Posteroanterior roentgenogram. Numerous small miliary or nodular shadows scattered throughout both lungs, but most obvious in the lower part. A single large nodular lesion is present below the right hilus (**arrow**). This type of metastasis is characteristic of papillary and follicular adenocarcinomas. These lesions may remain stationary for years. The trachea is displaced to the left by the thyroid neoplasm (**a**).

(Case *continued* in Figure 24.)

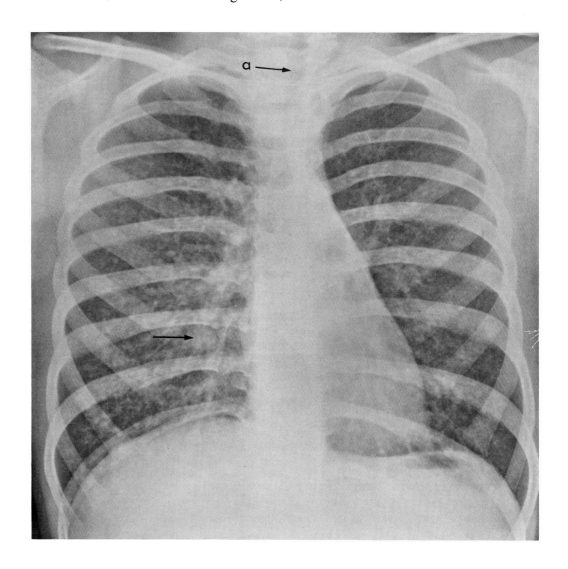

Figure 24.—Metastasis to the lung from thyroid papillary adenocarcinoma.

Posteroanterior roentgenogram. Same case as in Figure 23, 8 years later, after treatment by thyroidectomy and radioactive iodine. There is no visible evidence of neoplasm in the lungs, and the trachea is in the midline. Thyroidectomy increases the uptake of radioactive iodine by the metastasis.

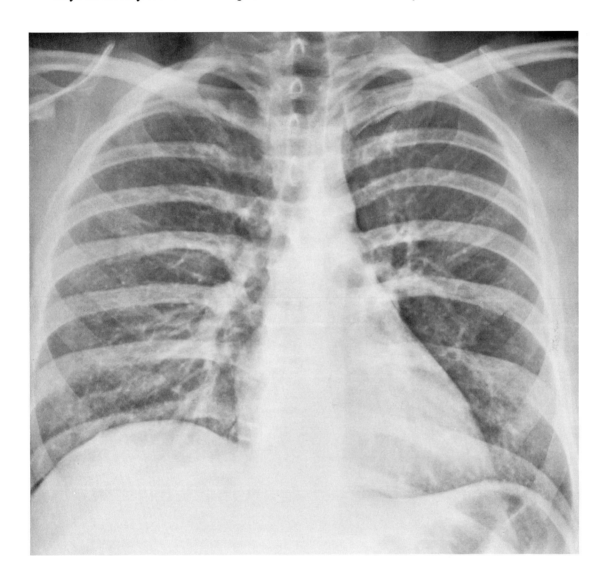

Figure 24 · Carcinoma: Pulmonary Metastases / 67

Figure 25.—Metastasis to the lung from a mixed papillary and follicular, predominantly papillary, adenocarcinoma of the thyroid.

Posteroanterior roentgenogram, demonstrating accentuated linear shadows of the lungs with miliary, indistinct, sometimes conglomerate shadows, seen almost exclusively in the lower two thirds of the lungs. The vessels are less distinct than normal because of adjacent metastatic growths.

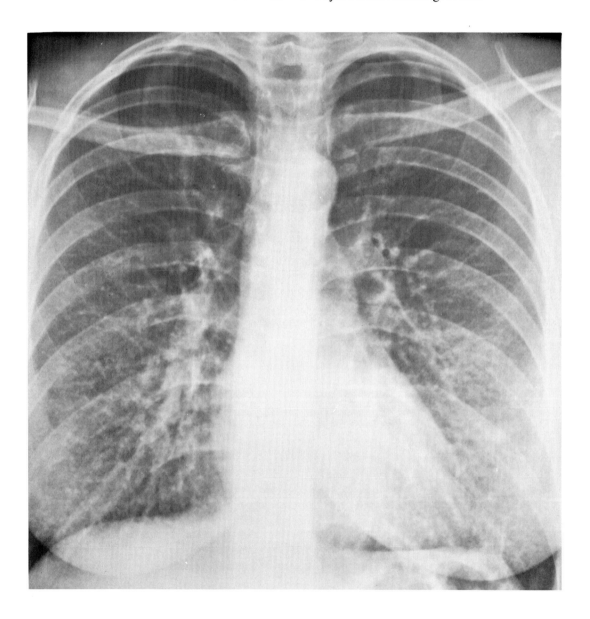

Figure 26.—Metastatsis to the lung from papillary adenocarcinoma of the thyroid.

Posteroanterior roentgenogram, demonstrating nodular lesions that are considerably larger than in the preceding cases. They are larger and more numerous in the lower part of the lungs. Some appear to have cavities, with air in the center of the lesions.

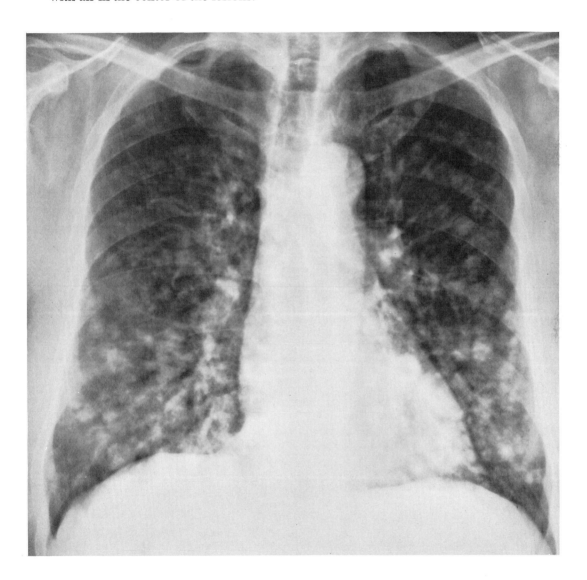

Figure 26 · Carcinoma: Pulmonary Metastases / 69

Figure 27.—Metastasis to bone from a follicular carcinoma of the thyroid.

Anteroposterior roentgenogram, showing a large, oval destructive lesion that involves the neck, lesser trochanter and adjacent shaft. The lesion has caused enlargement of the lesser trochanter through periosteal new bone formation, resulting in a new cortex. It has broken through the cortex and extended into the soft tissues. Coarse septa are visible. The lateral border consists of sclerotid reactive bone.

After this examination, the lesion was treated by external irradiation.

(Case *continued* in Figures 28 and 29.)

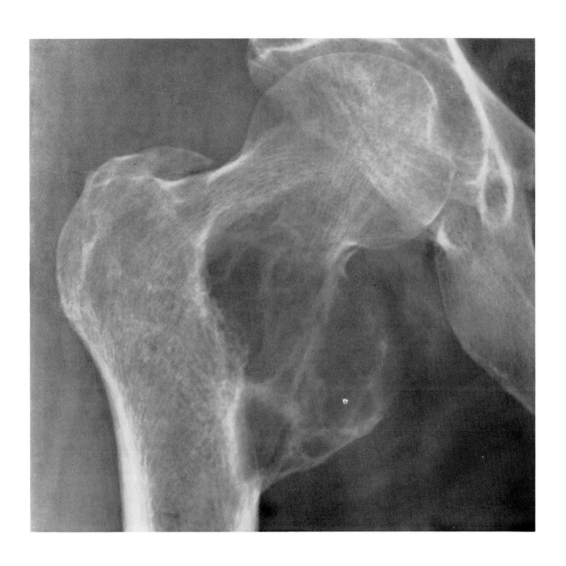

Figure 27 · Carcinoma: Bone Metastases / 71

Figure 28.—Metastasis to bone from thyroid carcinoma, with sarcomatous degeneration.

Same case as in Figure 27. The anteroposterior roentgenogram was obtained 10 years after roentgen therapy of the metastatic adenocarcinoma. A malignant process has completely destroyed the neck of the femur and extended into the head and along the shaft. No periosteal new bone is evident. A large, sharply demarcated, oval soft tissue mass is visible medial to the femur (**arrows**) where the cortex has been destroyed (**a**). Another lobulated soft tissue mass is seen above the greater trochanter which has been partially destroyed (**b**).

The leg and part of the pelvis were amputated, barium was injected into the major arteries, and transverse sections were made. Figure 29 shows a roentgenogram of one of these sections.

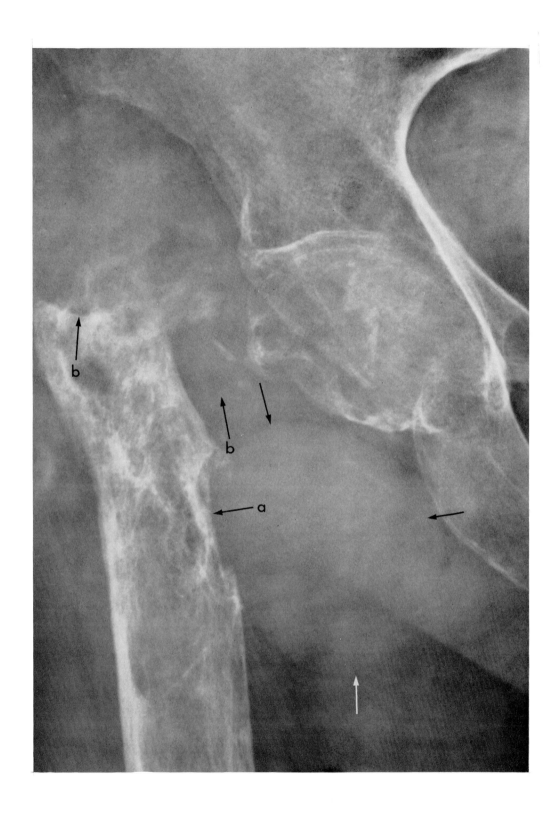

Figure 28 · Carcinoma: Bone Metastases / 73

Figure 29.—Roentgen-ray treated metastatic adenocarcinoma from the thyroid gland, with sarcomatous degeneration.

Same case as in Figures 27 and 28. This is a roentgenogram of one of the transverse sections of the amputated leg 10 years after roentgen treatment. The destroyed neck (**arrow**), shaft (**a**) and head (**b**) of the femur are visible. A spherical, sharply demarcated soft tissue mass, which is surrounded by opaque material from the arteriogram performed on the specimen, is seen medially (**c**). It communicates with similar tissue that has replaced the femoral neck. This was metastatic follicular adenocarcinoma. Another larger lobulated soft tissue mass involves the greater trochanter and neck of the femur and extends a considerable distance from bone (**d**). This was a fibrosarcoma, considered to be radiation-induced.

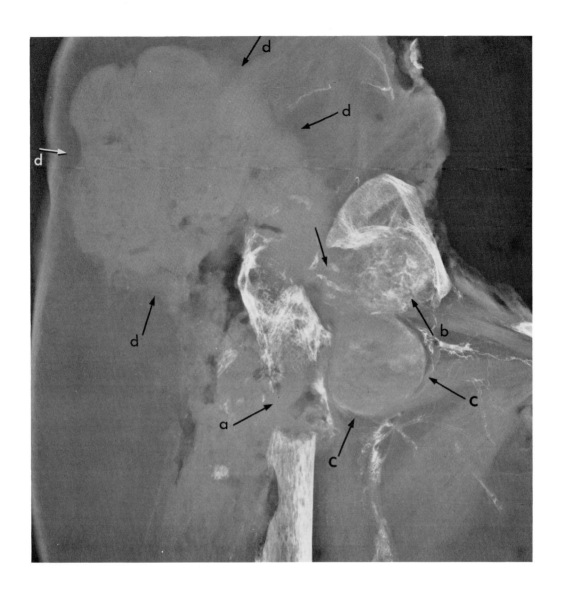

Figure 29 · Carcinoma: Bone Metastases / 75

Figure 30.—Metastases to the spine from adenocarcinoma of the thyroid.

A, anteroposterior roentgenogram of the lower thoracic spine, showing involvement by metastatic follicular adenocarcinoma of the thyroid gland. The ninth (**x**), tenth, and eleventh thoracic vertebral bodies are partially destroyed, as are the transverse processes and lamina of the tenth and eleventh vertebrae. Destruction is also seen in the adjacent tenth ribs (**y**). The intervertebral disk between the ninth and tenth vertebral bodies is narrowed (**a**). A lobulated soft tissue mass has spread in the soft tissues to the left of the spine (**b**). A smaller soft tissue mass is located to the right of the eleventh vertebra (**c**).

These lesions demonstrate characteristic features of thyroid metastasis to the bone. They are almost exclusively lytic except for small segments of sclerosis adjacent to the ninth intervertebral disk; they cross joints and intervertebral disks to involve the adjacent bones and extend into the soft tissues.

B, papillary adenocarcinoma of the thyroid metastatic to a thoracic vertebral body. This lateral roentgenogram of the lumbar spine shows a lytic lesion of the anterior two thirds of a vertebral body (**arrows**). The margins of the neoplasm are ill defined, and no evidence of reactive bone formation is evident. A nucleus pulposus has herniated into the lower end of the vertebra (**a**), possibly the result of weakened bone from the neoplasm.

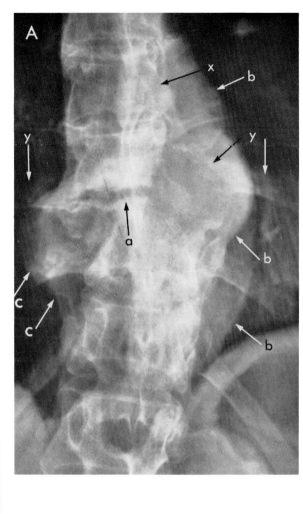

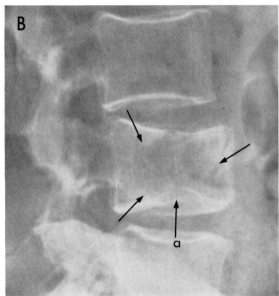

Figure 30 · Carcinoma: Bone Metastases / 77

Figure 31.—Thyroid acropachy.

The patient had previously been treated for Graves' disease and had exophthalmos, pretibial myxedema and clubbing of the fingers. The patient was maintained at a euthyroid level medically.

Posteroanterior roentgenogram of the hand. The horizontal line is an artifact. Clubbing of the soft tissues of the fingers is not well demonstrated. Periosteal new bone is best demonstrated along the ulnar border of the fifth metacarpal and, to a lesser extent, along the radial side of the first metacarpal. The radial side of the distal second metacarpal shaft is thickened distally. Additional periosteal thickening is present along the shafts of the second, fourth and fifth proximal phalanges (**arrows**). Typical localized soft tissue swellings are located adjacent to the areas of periosteal reaction.

The periosteal bone characteristically involves the midshafts of the metacarpals and phalanges. The new bone is often spiculated and at right angles to the shaft.

(*Continued* in Figure 32.)

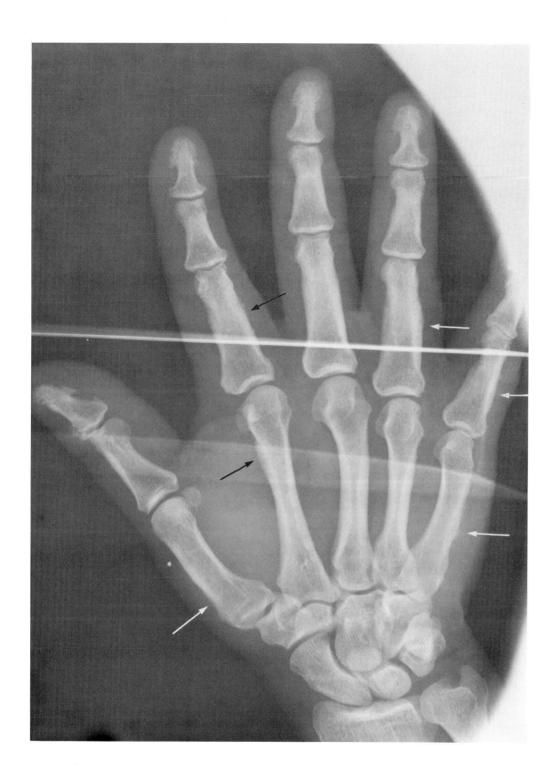

Figure 31 · Acropachy / 79

Figure 32.—Thyroid acropachy.

Same case as in Figure 31.

A, dorsoplantar roentgenogram of the left foot, demonstrating a thick first metatarsal cortex and adjacent soft tissue swelling (**arrows**).

B (same patient as in *A*), anteroposterior roentgenogram of the distal leg. Periosteal new bone has formed adjacent to the lateral cortical margin of the fibula (**arrows**). The layers of new bone are parallel to the original cortex and separated from it by a poorly defined dark line (**a**). The overlying skin is markedly thickened and dense (**b**).

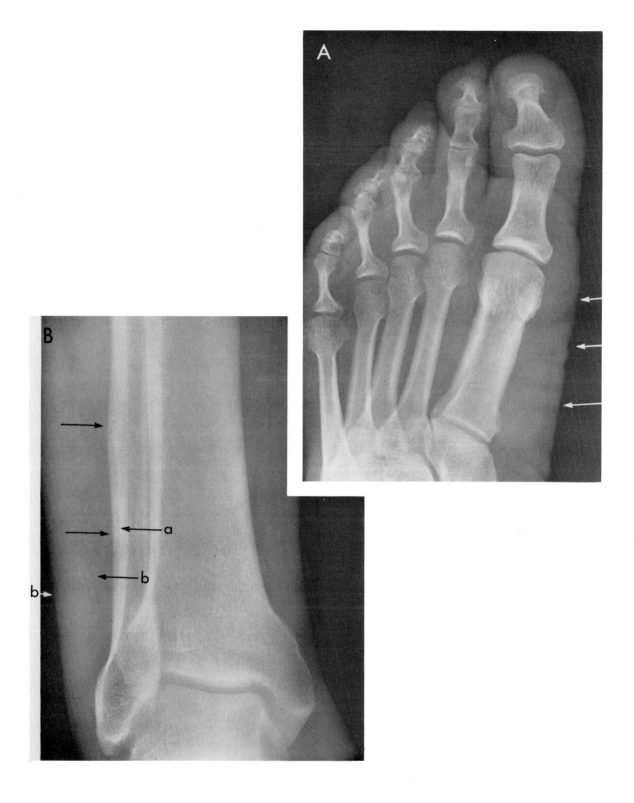

Figure 32 · Acropachy / 81

PART 3

The Parathyroid Glands

Neoplasms of the Parathyroid Glands

CLINICALLY DETECTABLE, nonfunctioning tumors or cysts of the parathyroid glands are uncommon. Oxyphil adenomas develop with advancing age and may represent an involuted chief cell adenoma. Cysts are generally the result of degeneration and are usually too small to be seen grossly or to be palpable. They usually arise from the inferior parathyroid glands and rarely produce symptoms from pressure on adjacent tissues. Primary nonfunctional carcinomas have been reported, but with more than half of carcinomas, hyperparathyroidism is present. Metastatic carcinoma not infrequently involves parathyroid tissue in cases of extensive carcinomatosis.

This discussion will be concerned mainly with functioning neoplasms of the parathyroid glands, since their diagnosis is usually established on the basis of metabolic and structural changes produced by an excess of parathyroid hormone. Often the parathyroid neoplasm is not palpable. A mass that is felt in the neck may not represent a tumor of the parathyroid gland, since in more than one fourth of our patients, parathyroid adenoma and an adenoma or carcinoma of the thyroid gland are present simultaneously.

HYPERPARATHYROIDISM

Parathyroid hormone is a polypeptide that is important in maintaining homeostasis of calcium and phosphorus in the plasma. The only stimulus proved to produce the hormone is a low plasma calcium content; elevated levels of calcium inhibit its production. It has two main direct and independent actions: (1) resorption of bone matrix by osteoclasts, thus elevating the plasma calcium content; (2) decreasing reabsorption of phosphate by the proximal tubules of the kidney, thus increasing urinary excretion of phosphorus and decreasing plasma phosphorus content. Other subsidiary actions of the hormone include the increased intestinal absorption of calcium, increased urinary excretion of magnesium and the decreased renal clearance of calcium.[1]

Hyperparathyroidism may cause disturbances of the urinary tract and skeletal system; it may give rise to symptoms of resultant acute hypercalcemia, or it may be present without evident symptoms. The evidence of urinary tract disturbances consists of hyposthenuria, polyuria, nocturia, poly-

---

[1] Jackson, W. P. U.: *Calcium Metabolism and Bone Disease* (London: Edward Arnold, Ltd., 1967).

dipsia and dehydration, most commonly observed in patients with severe hypercalcemia. The most common urinary tract complications are nephrolithiasis, pyelonephritis and nephrocalcinosis. Skeletal involvement may first be manifested by fractures with little or no trauma, but rarely by bone pain and tenderness. Localized expansion, bending or fracture may cause bone deformities.

The clinical symptoms of acute hypercalcemia are anorexia, nausea, vomiting, constipation, abdominal distention, thirst, nocturia, polyuria, weakness and, when the serum calcium level is exceedingly high, lethargy, somnolence or psychosis. Peptic ulcer is extremely common in patients with hyperparathyroidism.

The keystone of diagnosis is hypercalcemia, often of mild degree. Hypophosphatemia is found in about 40% of cases. Hyperphosphaturia is uniformly present.

Acute pancreatitis develops in some patients with hyperparathyroidism. Associated with hyperparathyroidism may be adenomas of several other endocrine glands, a condition called endocrine adenomatosis. The glands most commonly involved are the pancreatic islets, pituitary and parathyroids. Adenomas of the adrenal cortex and thyroid gland as well as tumors of the bronchi, multiple lipomatous tumors and other endocrine and nonendocrine tumors may be present. The pituitary adenomas may be chromophobe or eosinophilic and may be associated with acromegaly. Pancreatic islet cell tumors may secrete ulcerogenic hormone, producing the Zollinger-Ellison syndrome (see Part 4, The Pancreas), or nonulcerogenic hormone, inducing hyperinsulinism and hypoglycemia. Adrenal tumors may cause Cushing's syndrome, which is familial and is transmitted in a dominant manner.[2]

Hyperparathyroidism is rare in children younger than 10 years but, when present, may be familial. In young children, bone lesions are much more common than are renal calculi or nephrocalcinosis.

INCIDENCE; AGE; SEX.—It has been stated that 5% of all renal calculi are associated with hyperparathyroidism. Although hyperparathyroidism may develop at any time, it is usually seen between the ages of 30 and 60, being uncommon in children. Some large series report an equal sex incidence, but the accumulated experience indicates that hyperparathyroidism occurs three times more often in females than in males.

PATHOLOGIC CHANGES.—Neoplasms of the parathyroid glands may be classified into four main groups in order of incidence. About 80% are *adenomatous,* occasionally more than one adenoma being present. The adenoma may be smooth or lobulated, is encapsulated and is rimmed by

---

[2] Pyrah, L. N., *et al.*: Primary hyperparathyroidism, Brit. J. Surg. 53:245, April, 1966.

normal parathyroid tissue. It may contain calcium, cysts or fibrous scars. The chief cell is usually the predominant cell. In the *wasserhelle* adenomas, the cells are large and clear and rarely are there oxyphil cells, some of which do not produce hyperparathyroidism. All three cells may be seen in mixed-cell adenomas. The chief cell adenomas are the more common, followed next by mixed-cell adenomas.

Primary *wasserhelle* (water-clear) cell hyperplasia appears in 5–10% of cases. All parathyroid glands are enlarged unequally and are often lobulated. Two enlarged glands may coalesce to form a single mass. The cells are large and clear. They are usually uniformly present throughout the gland.

Primary *chief cell* hyperplasia occurs in 4–8% of cases. All glands are irregular or nodular and enlarged, but vary greatly in size and are usually smaller than water-clear hyperplasia. The upper glands are usually of normal parathyroid size. Histologically, the tumor may consist of a mass of nodules without a rim of normal parathyroid tissue. Adjacent nodules to some tumors may contain chief cells, large clear cells or oxyphil cells. Primary chief cell hyperplasia is present in patients with endocrine adenomatosis.

Carcinoma in parathyroid glands is uncommon, varying from 0.5 to 2.0% in hyperparathyroidism. The cytologic study may show similarities to benign adenomas, but malignancy is inferred because of invasion of surrounding tissue or a distant metastasis. Some apparently benign adenomas contain atypical cells that suggest a malignant process.[3]

Skeletal system.—Osteitis fibrosa cystica generalisata affects the entire skeleton. The earliest and most severe lesions appear in regions where normal bone production and the invariably associated bone destruction or remodeling occur most rapidly. In children, some of the most pronounced changes are in the metaphyses adjoining the growth plate, where calcified cartilage is replaced by primitive bone, which in turn undergoes remodeling through the mechanism of osteoclastic resorption and surface accretion. In both adult and child, early lesions usually appear along the periosteal surface of the cortex, particularly at the point of tendinous or ligamentous attachments. Sites of injury, mechanical pressure or tension, with osteoclastic bone destruction and osteoblastic repair, appear to be more sensitive to the parathyroid hormone.

The well-developed histologic lesion is caused by osteoclastic resorption of bone, associated with reparative fibrosis and formation of poorly calcified

---

[3] Castleman, B.: Tumors of the Parathyroid Glands, in *Atlas of Tumor Pathology*, Sect. IV, fasc. 15 (Washington, D.C.: Armed Forces Institute of Pathology, 1952); Netter, F. H.: Endocrine System and Selected Metabolic Diseases, in *Ciba Collection of Medical Illustrations* (Summit, N. J.: Ciba Pharmaceutical Products, Inc., 1965), Vol. 4; Danowski, T. S.: *Clinical Endocrinology* (Baltimore: Williams & Wilkins Company, 1962), Vol. 3.

immature new bone. The compact, cortical bone is replaced by spongy bone. Localized accumulations of fibrous tissue and giant cells, called "brown tumors," may produce expansion of bone similar to giant cell and other benign tumors. Brown tumors undergoing necrosis and liquefaction produce cysts.

Urinary tract.—Renal calculi containing calcium phosphate or calcium oxalate are present in about three fourths of the patients. Usually, one or more calculi are found in the calyces or pelvis. Much less commonly, small calculi (nephrocalcinosis) are found in the distal tubules or, even less often, in the loop of Henle or the collecting tubules and surrounding renal tissue (Fig. 36). Nephrocalcinosis is identified much more frequently on histologic examination than on roentgenographic. Kidneys with both renal calculi and nephrocalcinosis are rare. The parenchymal changes consist of various degrees of tubular damage and cellular tubular casts in addition to concretions. Secondary effects are the result of hydronephrosis, pyelonephritis and pyonephrosis. In patients with roentgenographically visible nephrocalcinosis, skeletal lesions are usually visible on the roentgenograms, whereas in most patients with renal calculi the bones appear to be normal.

ROENTGEN CHANGES.[4]—Usually, the skeleton is less dense than normal; however, the density is often normal or, rarely, increased. In other instances, localized areas of diminished and increased density in the same bone may be present.

Cortical erosion.—In advanced hyperparathyroidism, all of the cortical surfaces may be involved. In certain sites of predilection, however, cortical erosion may be visible before other manifestations of the disease. The sites most frequently involved are the lateral (radial) aspect of the middle phalanges of the hands and the tufts of the distal phalanges (Figs. 37 and 38). Other regions where early subperiosteal cortical erosion may be present are the articulations of the distal end of the clavicle, the symphysis pubis (Fig. 41) and the sacroiliac joints. Similar erosions may be noted in the lamina dura (the cortical bone surrounding the root of the tooth; see Fig. 39, *A*), the calcaneal tendon insertions at the plantar or Achilles surfaces, the medial aspect of the proximal end of the tibia (Fig. 40, *A*), the ischial tuberosities, the greater and lesser trochanters, the crests of the ilia and the posterior superior margins of the third and fourth or lower ribs.

The roentgenographic appearance of the subperiosteal cortical erosion is the same in different bones. The normal smooth outer surface of the cortex at first loses its sharp demarcation from the surrounding soft tissues. Later,

---

[4] Steinbach, H. L., *et al.*: Primary hyperparathyroidism: A correlation of roentgen, clinical, and pathologic features, Am. J. Roentgenol. 86:329, August, 1961.

areas of destruction alternating with normal-appearing bone may produce spicules perpendicular to the cortical surface. In tubular bones, these changes are associated with vertical striations of the middle and deeper layers of the cortex caused by widening of the haversian canals, the longitudinal spaces enclosing the blood vessels and surrounding connective tissue. Such typical subperiosteal resorption occurs in no other disease.

Localized destructive lesions.—Also known as brown tumors, these are frequently found in the jaws or facial bones, but may be present in any part of the skeleton (Fig. 42, *B*). In the shaft of a long bone, they may be eccentric. They are usually sharply demarcated and may expand the cortex. A single lesion of one bone, or many lesions involving several bones, may be present. The brown tumors heal after removal of the parathyroid tumor or after local radiation therapy or curettage. Some undergo cystic degeneration, persisting as defects in the bone after the primary disease has been cured. The cystic lesions do not differ roentgenographically from the tumors and they can be recognized only by their failure to heal after treatment.

In a few cases of proved hyperparathyroidism, a mottled skull or a large destructive lesion was seen, without subperiosteal resorption.

Calcification of soft tissues.—Calcification of the soft tissues, other than the kidneys or articular cartilages, is uncommon except when severe kidney disease is present. Chondrocalcinosis, seen in about 18% of our patients, was almost as common as the bone lesions. It may be present in the absence of bone disease. It is well seen in the menisci and articular cartilage of the knees (Fig. 43, *A*), in the triangular and articular cartilages of the wrists (Fig. 42, *C* and *D*) and in the articular cartilage of the shoulders, hips and symphysis pubis (Fig. 43, *B*) and of other joints.

Tumor identification.—When the parathyroid tumor is large, it may displace the trachea or esophagus (Fig. 33). Benign or malignant thyroid neoplasms in these patients may, however, also displace these structures. Selective angiography may be employed to demonstrate the neoplasm, best accomplished by injecting contrast medium into the thyrocervical trunk and filling the inferior thyroid artery (Fig. 34). Substernal neoplasms may be supplied by the internal mammary artery. If inferior thyroid artery injection is not successful, the internal mammary vessels should be investigated. The site of the parathyroid adenoma may be diagnosed by a displacement or distortion of the inferior thyroid artery or by abnormal vessels with a vascular blush within the tumor. Tumors of the thyroid gland may appear similar to those of the parathyroid glands.[5]

---

[5] Newton, T. H., and Eisenberg, E.: Angiography of parathyroid adenomas, Radiology 86:843, May, 1966.

Other diseases, such as renal failure, osteomalacia and pseudohypoparathyroidism, which produce low serum calcium levels stimulate the parathyroids to produce an excess of parathyroid hormone. The resultant roentgen appearance of the skeleton is often similar except for a lower incidence of brown tumors and cysts and absence of chondrocalcinosis. With severe renal failure, areas of the bone are often dense, particularly the metaphyses and regions beneath the end-plates of the vertebrae. The vertebral bands are characteristic of renal failure and have been called the "rugger jersey" sign. The parathyroid glands are usually hyperplastic with secondary hyperplasia, but one or more may form an autonomous adenoma with function independent of stimulus from hypocalcemia. With renal failure and particularly after renal dialysis, calcific deposits often form in the capsules of tendons and ligaments of joints. These deposits may appear as faint streaks of calcium or larger, irregular amorphous masses. They are often seen around the joints of the fingers but may be present around the larger joints. The calcified regions may be painful. The deposits are different from those in patients with primary hyperparathyroidism, in which calcification of articular cartilage and fibrocartilage is frequently observed.

Severe renal failure with secondary hyperparathyroidism in young children may initially be manifested as rickets, with failure of calcification of the epiphyseal cartilage and the zone of provisional calcification. On the roentgenogram, the space between the epiphysis and metaphysis appears to be wider than normal; this is best seen in the knees and the distal end of the radius and ulna.

As the renal disease progresses, the signs of rickets may tend to regress, and resorption of bone in the metaphysis beneath the zone of provisional calcification is increased. Associated with this resorption, the epiphyses may be slipped (fractures through the weakened area beneath the zone of provisional calcification). Frequently, this slipping involves the proximal femoral and humeral epiphyses; less often, the metacarpal and metatarsal epiphyses are affected. When roentgen signs of both rickets and hyperparathyroidism are apparent in childhood, the diagnosis of renal failure may be suspected.

Pseudohyperparathyroidism is a condition in which the kidneys, and perhaps other tissues, respond inadequately to normal or excessive amounts of parathyroid hormone. This disease is a familial one. The patients are usually of short stature, and calcification or ossification is demonstrable in the soft tissues. The serum calcium content is low and phosphate level high, leading to an excess of secretion of parathyroid hormone. As a result, the roentgenograms show evidence of osteitis fibrosa, as described previously, and slipped epiphyses. The parathyroid glands are often hyperplastic.

Figure 33.—Identifying the parathyroid tumor.

A, anteroposterior view, showing displacement of the esophagus and trachea to the right and compression of the trachea by a huge parathyroid adenoma (**arrows**).

B, anteroposterior view, showing the esophagus displaced to the right by a large left adenoma (**arrows**). The normal appearance of the trachea, which lies in front of the esophagus, indicates that the tumor lies posteriorly.

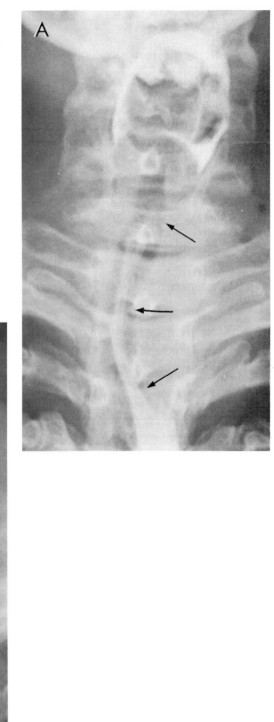

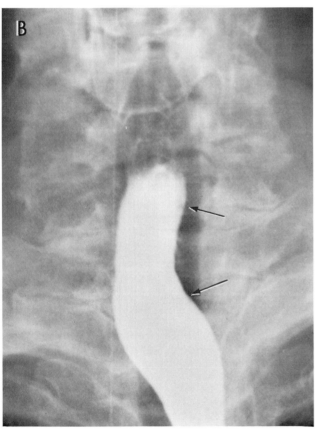

Figure 33 · Parathyroid Tumor: Identification / 93

Figure 34.—Identifying the parathyroid tumor.

A, selective angiography, with injection into the internal mammary artery (**a**). This early roentgenogram shows a large branch of the artery (**b**) pursuing a tortuous course to an oval mass in the anterior mediastinum. The vessel surrounds the parathyroid adenoma and gives off small branches to the tumor (**c**).

This patient had no symptoms but was found to have hypercalcemia on routine physical examination. Previous neck surgery had not revealed a tumor. Selective angiography is also useful in identifying parathyroid neoplasms in the neck.

B (same patient as in *A*), later roentgenogram after same injection of contrast medium. The contrast medium is in the arteries and capillaries of this very vascular tumor, causing it to be opaque (**d**). Two large veins converge (**e**) to form one vessel entering the left innominate vein (**f**).

The adenoma is in the anterior mediastinum which is the usual location of aberrant parathyroids.

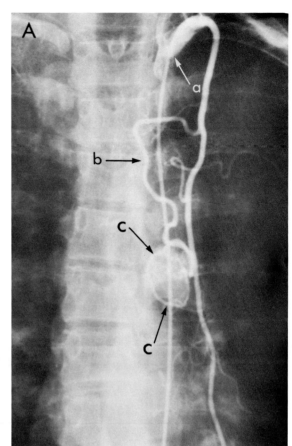

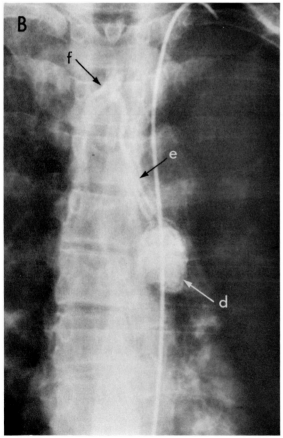

Figure 34 · Parathyroid Tumor: Identification / 95

Figure 35.—Mediastinal parathyroid carcinoma.

The patient had a history of repeated renal calculi. There were no complaints referable to the chest.

A, posteroanterior routine examination of the chest: A sharply demarcated mass is overlying the right hilus (**arrows**).

B, oblique view of the chest: There is slight posterior displacement of the esophagus (**arrow**). Part of the tumor is visible to the right of the esophagus (**a**).

C, lateral view of the chest: No abnormalities are apparent except for slight posterior displacement of the esophagus (**arrow**).

Figure 35, courtesy of Dr. D. J. Stephenson, Lakewood, Colo.

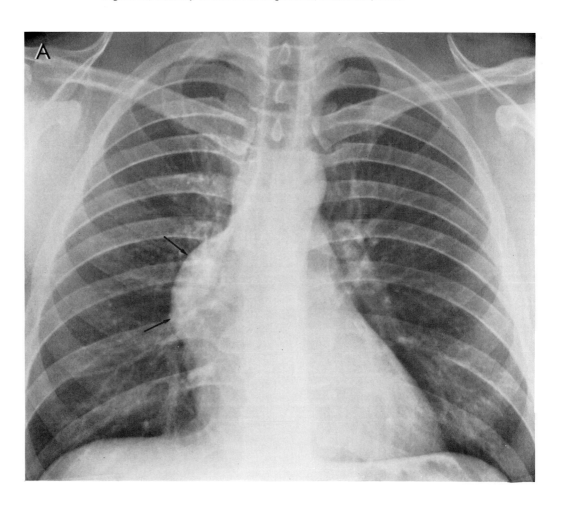

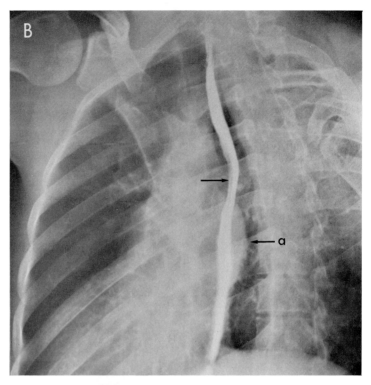

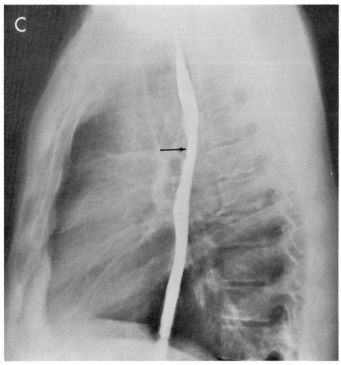

Figure 35 · Mediastinal Parathyroid Carcinoma / 97

Figure 36.—Nephrocalcinosis in hyperparathyroidism.

Anteroposterior view: Numerous calcifications of various sizes are distributed throughout the medullary substance of the kidneys. Some are concentrated in the region of the renal papillae (**a**). The cortex and the kidneys, over all, are slightly diminished in size (**b**). Other diseases associated with hypercalcemia induce a similar response in the kidneys.

Nephrocalcinosis is an unusual finding in hyperparathyroidism. When it is present, there are almost always bone lesions and the parathyroid adenoma is large. Most patients with hyperparathyroidism have renal calculi lying in the calices, pelvis, ureter or bladder that are singular or multiple, unilateral or bilateral. They are similar to renal calculi that form without hyperparathyroidism. These patients usually do not have skeletal lesions and their parathyroid lesion tends to be small.

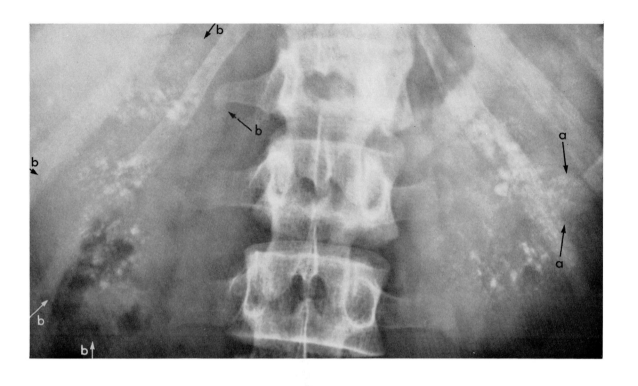

Figure 36 · Hyperparathyroidism: Nephrocalcinosis / 99

Figure 37.—Subperiosteal resorption of bone in hyperparathyroidism.

A, posteroanterior projection, revealing extensive osteitis fibrosa involving the bones of the hand. The middle phalanges show subperiosteal resorption of the outer cortical margin (**a**). The normally smooth cortex is replaced by a rough spiculated surface and the phalanx is narrow. This is seen best on the side of the phalanges facing the thumb. Slight resorption is also present in the other phalanges and ulnar side of the third, fourth and fifth metacarpal heads (**b**).

The tufts of all distal phalanges have been partially resorbed (**c**). There are discrete destructive lesions of the third middle, fourth proximal and first distal phalanges (**d**). Whether these lesions are brown tumors or cysts is impossible to tell until healing has taken place. The bones are demineralized and vertical striations are prominent. The second proximal phalanx has a dense distal portion (**e**) which represents a healed brown tumor. This is sometimes seen in the presence of active disease elsewhere.

B (same patient as in *A*), this roentgenogram, exposed as in *A*, obtained several months after a parathyroid adenoma was removed, shows evidence of healing. The cortical bone has been reconstituted in all areas previously affected by subperiosteal resorption. There is actually an overgrowth of bone into the capsular attachments surrounding the joints, as seen at the proximal ends of the second and third middle phalanges and heads of the second and third metacarpals (**e**). The radiolucent lesions of the third middle and fourth proximal phalanges have not filled in (**d**), indicating that they were cysts.

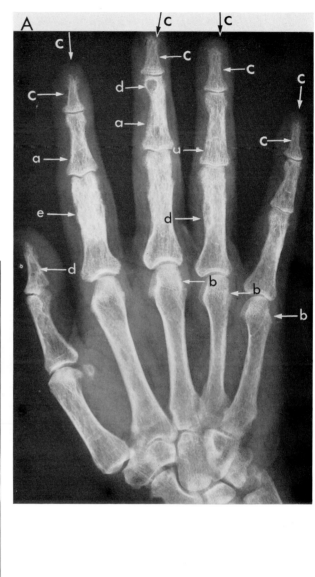

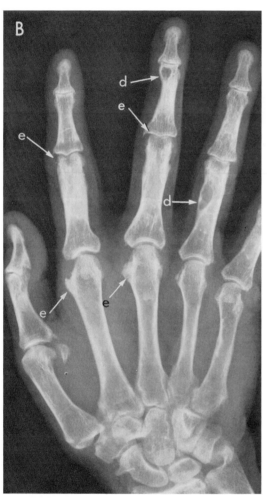

Figure 37 · Hyperparathyroidism: Bone Resorption / 101

Figure 38.—Subperiosteal resorption of bone in hyperparathyroidism.

A, in this posteroanterior exposure of a patient with osteitis fibrosa, the over-all density of the bones is normal. Subperiosteal cortical resorption is limited to the second, third and fourth middle phalanges, primarily on the surface facing the thumb (**a**). A discrete larger defect is present in the middle phalanx (**b**). The shafts of the first, second and third distal phalanges show slight resorption (**c**).

B, anteroposterior view of the first toe, showing subperiosteal resorption of the medial cortex of the middle phalanx (**arrow**).

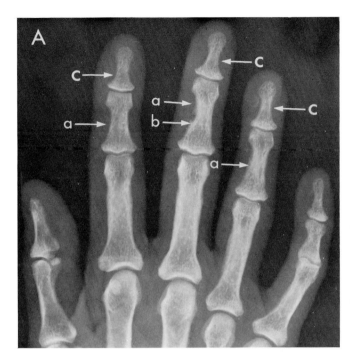

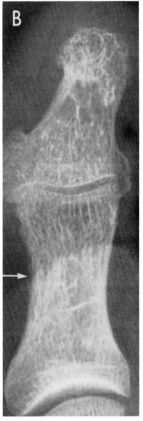

Figure 38 · Hyperparathyroidism: Bone Resorption / 103

Figure 39.—Skull and facial lesions of hyperparathyroidism (all figures from same patient).

A, magnified view of a destructive lesion of the maxilla (**a**). Two teeth have been exfoliated. The lamina dura, which is cortical bone surrounding the tooth, is absent (**b**).

B, lateral view, revealing mottled appearance of the skull caused by destructive lesions adjacent to areas of sclerosis. A larger discrete destructive focal lesion is present in the frontal bone (**arrow**). The lesions are most obvious in the outer third of the frontal and parietal bones.

C, lateral view, demonstrating healed lesions. The calvarium (**a**) and orbital plates (**b**) are more dense and thicker than normal. Persistent radiolucent defects (**c**) probably represent areas of cystic degeneration. A healing expanding lesion of the posterior maxilla is now visible as it becomes opacified (**d**); it was not seen on the original roentgenograms.

The patient also had a tumor of the pituitary (not demonstrated on the roentgenograms), an islet cell tumor with Zollinger-Ellison syndrome and chief cell adenomas of all four parathyroid glands.

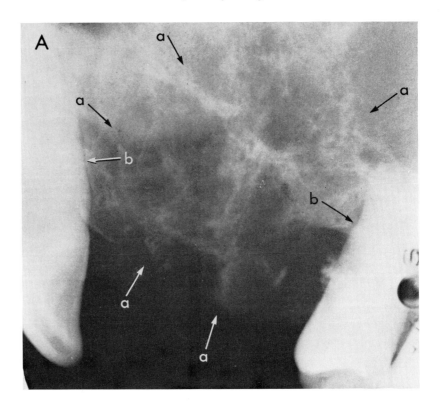

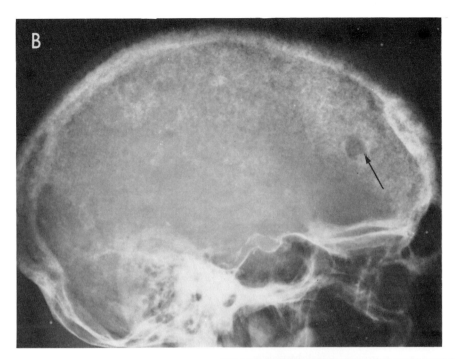

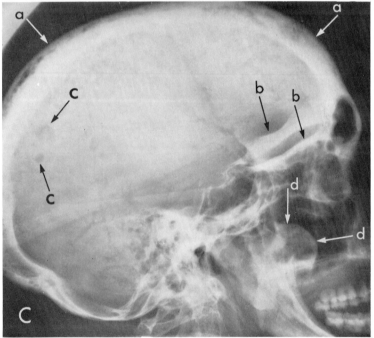

Figure 39 · Hyperparathyroidism: Skull and Face Lesions / 105

Figure 40.—Subperiosteal lesions of hyperparathyroidism.

A, anteroposterior view, revealing a destructive subperiosteal lesion of the proximal medial metaphysis of the tibia in the region of the insertion of tendons (**arrows**).

B, lateral projection, showing subperiosteal resorption of the calcaneus adjacent to the plantar fascial and muscle attachments (**arrow**). There is also some resorption of the upper posterior calcaneus adjacent to the insertion of the Achilles tendon.

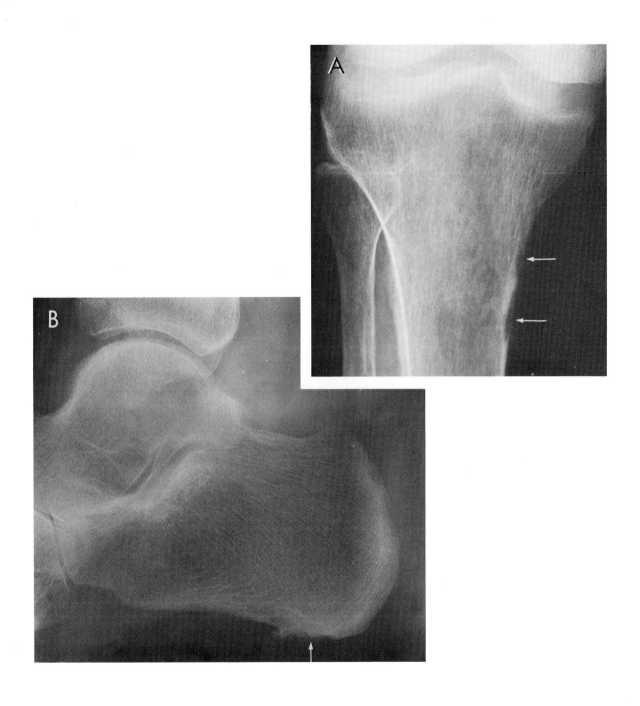

Figure 40 · **Hyperparathyroidism: Subperiosteal Lesions** / **107**

Figure 41.—Subperiosteal lesions of hyperparathyroidism.

A, anteroposterior view, revealing subperiosteal resorption of the ischium (**arrows**), seen best on the right side.

B, anteroposterior view after treatment. The irregular ischial cortex is beginning to fill in with new bone (**arrows**).

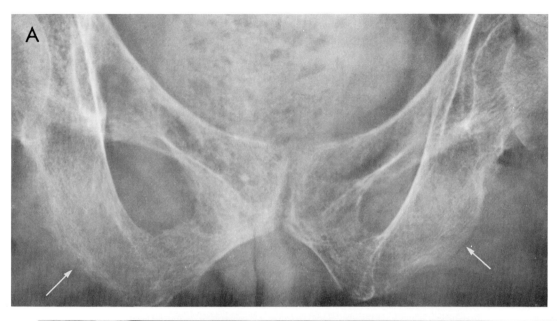

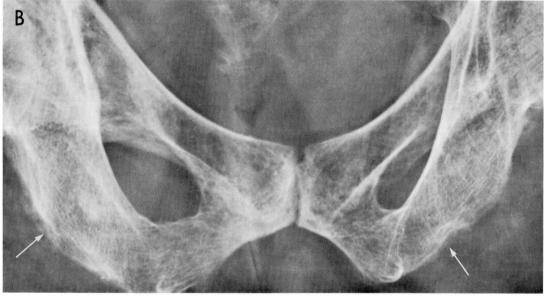

Figure 41 · Hyperparathyroidism: Subperiosteal Lesions / 109

Figure 42.—Localized destructive lesions of hyperparathyroidism.

A, anteroposterior view of the hip, revealing a sharply demarcated, multilocular lesion with a slightly sclerotic border involving the right acetabulum (**a**). Another lesion is in the neck of the right femur (**b**).

B (*B–D* from same patient), anteroposterior view, demonstrating brown tumors of the neck (**a**) and shaft (**b**) of the right femur. The upper lesion is trabeculated and involves only spongy bone. The lower lesion is centrally located and oval, with the long axis corresponding to that of the bone. The endosteal surface is eroded by the mass, producing a sharply defined border.

C, posteroanterior view of the right wrist. Calcified cartilage (chondrocalcinosis) involves the triangular cartilage of the wrist just distal to the ulna (**a**) and also the articular cartilage of the semilunare and triquetrum (**b**). A small destructive process involves the semilunare (**c**).

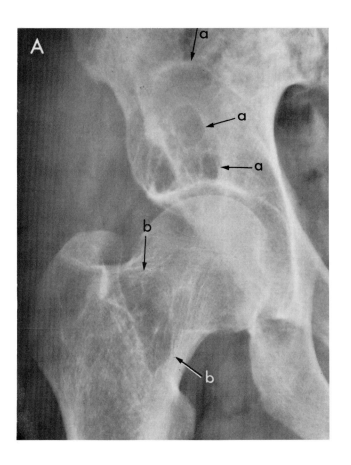

D, posteroanterior view of the left wrist. Chondrocalcinosis, barely demonstrable, is almost identical to that in the right wrist (**a** and **b**). The semilunare also has a destructive lesion (**c**). A healed sclerotic lesion is present in the distal radius (**d**) despite the active disease process elsewhere.

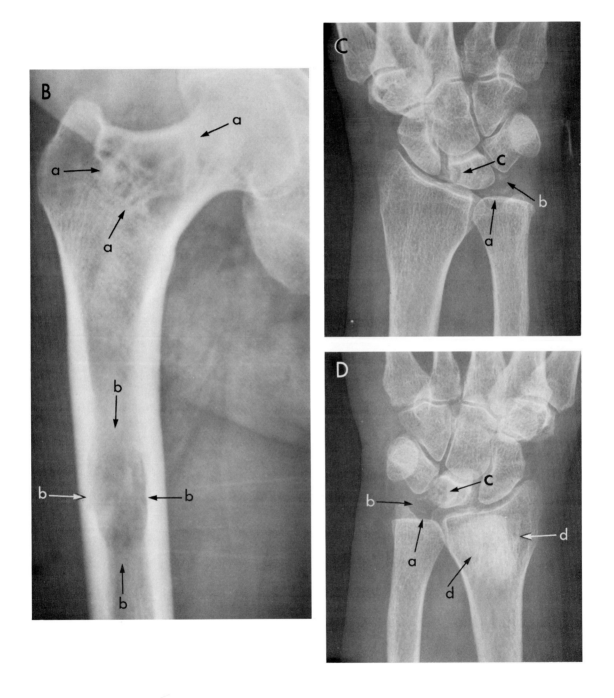

Figure 42 · **Hyperparathyroidism: Localized Bone Lesion** / **111**

Figure 43.—Chondrocalcinosis with hyperparathyroidism.

A, anteroposterior view, revealing chondrocalcinosis involving the menisci (**a**) and articular cartilages (**b**).

B, anteroposterior view, showing chondrocalcinosis of the hyaline articular cartilage of the hip (**a**) and the fibrocartilage of the symphysis pubis (**b**).

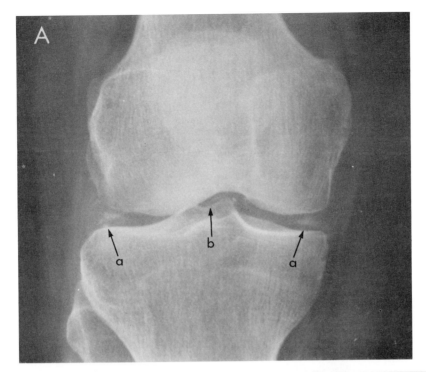

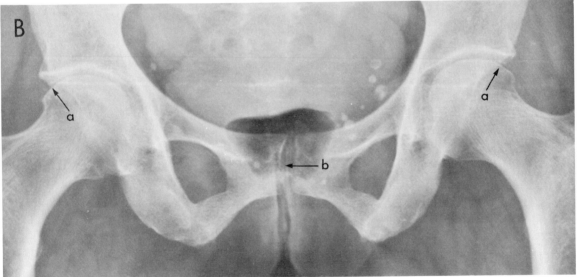

Figure 43 · Hyperparathyroidism: Chondrocalcinosis / 113

PART 4

The Pancreas

Manifestations of Pancreatic Lesions

CARCINOMA OF THE PANCREAS

CARCINOMA OF THE PANCREAS accounts for approximately 1% of all cancers. It is a disease of the aged, seen most frequently in the sixth, seventh and eighth decades of life. It is preponderant in males in a ratio of about 2:1.

PATHOLOGIC CHANGES.—The term carcinoma of the pancreas refers to malignant tumors arising from the exocrine ductal epithelium. Tumors that arise from the endocrine islets of Langerhans are specifically designated islet cell tumors. The carcinomas are most often of the scirrhous type. Invasion of surrounding structures is facilitated by the absence of a capsule around the pancreas. The rich lymphatic and vascular supply to the pancreatic bed facilitates regional metastasis. Metastatic growths are found most frequently in the regional nodes and liver. Perineural invasion occurs often and accounts for the frequency and severity of pain in patients with pancreatic carcinoma. Most pancreatic carcinomas are located in the head of the pancreas (60–70%); 20–30% are in the body of the pancreas, and 5–10% in the tail.

Because of their proximity to the ampulla of Vater and common bile duct, tumors in the head of the pancreas cause biliary symptoms relatively early in the course of the disease. Consequently, they are likely to be discovered while they are still small and before metastasis is widespread. Usually, the tumor extends to the medial margin of the duodenum, frequently invading its wall and narrowing the distal common bile duct and pancreatic duct. Stenosis or complete obstruction of the common bile duct, in turn, causes pronounced distention of the hepatobiliary tree and, frequently, of the gallbladder. The presence or absence of a distended gallbladder is unreliable, however, in distinguishing between obstructive jaundice caused by stone and that caused by tumor of the head of the pancreas. Cholecystitis is sometimes associated with tumor, preventing distention of the gallbladder. Conversely, fibrotic changes in the gallbladder may not be of sufficient magnitude to prevent its distention when obstructive jaundice is the result of a common duct stone.

Carcinomas of the body and tail are identical histologically to tumors arising in the head of the pancreas. Because of their location, they are frequently larger and more extensive than those arising in the head. Body and tail tumors may extend anteriorly to involve the stomach or transverse colon, invade posteriorly to involve the spine or extend by way of the retroperitoneal space superiorly or inferiorly.

CLINICAL FINDINGS.—Abdominal pain, jaundice and weight loss are the most frequent presenting symptoms of carcinoma of the head of the pancreas. Pain often precedes the jaundice, which is the initial symptom in 20–25% of patients. Intractable pruritus often accompanies jaundice. With carcinoma of the pancreatic body and tail, pain and loss of weight without jaundice are the most common symptoms. The pain, when characteristic, is usually dull and penetrating and radiates through to the back. It is usually intensified in the supine position, which results in pressure on the celiac plexus. For unknown reasons, multiple venous thromboses develop in some instances.

Because of the deep location of the pancreas, a palpable mass is rarely noted. Ascites, due to thrombosis or compression of the portal vein or of peritoneal metastasis, may be present.

Pancreatic carcinoma usually progresses rapidly, resulting in death in less than a year after the onset of symptoms.

ROENTGEN CHANGES.—By means of the conventional upper gastrointestinal series, accuracy in the diagnosis of pancreatic tumors has been estimated at 40–50%. Most missed diagnoses may be attributed to the unique location of the pancreas, which often permits considerable tumor growth before altered surroundings are detectable roentgenographically. Masses of the pancreas are primarily manifested by deformity and displacement of the barium-filled gastrointestinal tract. The roentgen findings vary, depending on the size and location of the lesion. Thus, with smaller tumors arising in any portion of the pancreas, there may be no evidence of abnormality on routine barium examination of the upper gastrointestinal tract. Larger tumors arising in the head of the pancreas may widen the duodenal loop or efface the duodenal mucosa along the medial margin of the loop (Figs. 44–46). The gastric antrum may be displaced forward and upward.

The stomach is the structure most frequently affected by masses arising in the pancreatic body and tail. Anterior displacement or localized impression on the body of the stomach may be seen only on lateral roentgenograms (Fig. 45, C). Lateral views should always be included in examinations of the upper gastrointestinal tract when a pancreatic mass is suspected. Displacement or distortion of the third and fourth portions of the duodenum (Fig. 44, B) and of the ligament of Treitz should also be sought.

Other structures that pancreatic cysts and tumors may involve are the transverse colon and splenic flexure, gastric fundus, distal esophagus, kidney and, rarely, the gallbladder.

Direct invasion of neighboring gut by pancreatic carcinoma is manifested roentgenographically by fixation of mucosal folds, filling defects within the gut lumen and ulceration or rigidity of the affected structure. When any of these changes is associated with a pancreatic mass, carcinoma rather than a cyst should be suspected. Their absence does not, however, exclude the diagnosis of carcinoma.

Advances in the roentgen diagnosis of pancreatic masses include hypotonic duodenography, arteriography and percutaneous transhepatic chol angiography. For hypotonic duodenography, duodenal atony is induced by an intramuscular injection of 60 mg of Probanthine. A catheter is then introduced into the proximal duodenum and barium and air are injected. The examination permits excellent demonstration of duodenal anatomy, unhindered by peristaltic activity (Fig. 57, C).

Arteriography in patients with pancreatic carcinoma may reveal displacement of vessels, arterial stenosis or obstruction and irregular, tortuous tumor vessels. Except for pancreatic cystadenomas and some islet cell tumors, a pronounced vascular blush is not noted in pancreatic neoplasms (Figs. 53, B and C; 57, D).

Percutaneous transhepatic cholangiography frequently helps to distinguish obstructive jaundice caused by tumor in the region of the ampulla of Vater from that caused by common bile duct stone. Obstruction by carcinoma of the head of the pancreas is typically manifested by extrinsic narrowing of the dilated lumen of the common bile duct (Fig. 57, B). The outline of the lumen is even and smooth. In contrast, calculi in the common duct are manifested by filling defects within the duct lumen, whose margins are sharply defined.

ISLET CELL TUMORS

The most common benign neoplasm of the pancreas is the islet cell adenoma. Lopez-Kruger and Dockerty[1] found 44 islet cell tumors in 10,314 consecutive autopsies. In 9,158 consecutive autopsies, Frantz[2] noted 24 benign islet cell adenomas. Howard et al.[3] reviewed 398 islet cell tumors reported in the literature of which 264 were associated with hyperinsulinism and 102 were not. No statement regarding hypoglycemia was noted in the remaining 32. Although these tumors can occur at any age from infancy to

[1] Lopez-Kruger, R., and Dockerty, M. G.: Tumors of the islets of Langerhans, Surg., Gynec. & Obst. 85:495, October, 1947.

[2] Frantz, V. K.: Tumors of the Pancreas, in *Atlas of Tumor Pathology*, Sect. VII, fasc. 27 and 28 (Washington, D.C.: Armed Forces Institute of Pathology, 1959).

[3] Howard, J. M., et al.: Hyperinsulinism and islet cell tumors of the pancreas with 398 recorded tumors, Internat. Abst. Surg. 90:417, May, 1950.

the eighth decade, most of those associated with hyperinsulinism were in patients between 35 and 60. No sex predilection was noted.

Non-insulin-producing islet cell tumors associated with the Zollinger-Ellison syndrome have been reported in increasing numbers since the syndrome was first described in 1955. At least 500 cases have been described in the literature, and undoubtedly many others have not been reported.

PATHOLOGIC CHANGES.—About 65% of islet cell tumors are found in the body and tail of the pancreas. Multiple adenomas constitute 10–15% of islet cell tumors. Rarely, the islet cell tumors may exist in ectopic foci of pancreatic tissue. The tumors are usually small (1–2 cm in diameter) and well circumscribed. Typically, they are encapsulated, firm nodules that compress the surrounding pancreatic substance by expansile growth. On histologic examination, the adenomatous cells closely resemble those of normal islets. Even the malignant lesions show little evidence of anaplasia, and their histologic appearance may give no clue to their biologic behavior. The diagnosis of islet cell carcinoma is not warranted in the absence of unmistakable metastasis or local invasion beyond the confines of the pancreas. Malignancy is found in approximately 10% of cases.

Non-beta cell tumors are frequently associated with the Zollinger-Ellison syndrome. These tumors produce a potent gastrin-like hormone, resulting in excessive gastric hypersecretion and a fulminating ulcer diathesis. In contrast to the insulin-producing beta cell tumors, about 60% of the tumors associated with the Zollinger-Ellison syndrome are malignant. Among the benign lesions producing the Zollinger-Ellison syndrome, 30% are adenomas and 10% show islet cell hyperplasia. Gastric secretagogue is produced in multiple sites in approximately 55% of these tumors. As with the insulin-secreting pancreatic tumors, the histologic evaluation of the tumor is not a reliable criterion of its biologic behavior. The regional lymph nodes are the most commonly affected extrapancreatic site. Next in frequency are local invasion into peripancreatic tissues and metastasis to the liver.

Non-beta cell tumors may be associated with severe diarrhea, without gastric hypersecretion or peptic ulceration.

CLINICAL FINDINGS.—Insulin-producing adenomas are frequently suspected clinically because of signs and symptoms of hypoglycemia. The designation Whipple's triad applies to the characteristic clinical manifestations that these pancreatic lesions produce. The triad consists of: (1) spontaneous hypoglycemia associated with such central nervous system manifestations as confusion, stupor and loss of consciousness, clearly related to fasting or exercise; (2) repeated blood sugar levels below 50 mg/100 ml, and (3) relief of symptoms when glucose is administered parenterally. Since the symptoms of excessive insulin secretion appear with fasting, early-morning attacks are common. The output of insulin by islet cell tumors is not subject to normal physiologic control; therefore attacks of symptoms are not related to previous carbohydrate intake. Excessive activity of the sympathetic nervous system, as manifested by sweating, nausea, chills and rapid pulse, is usually associated with the hypoglycemic episodes.

The original triad described by Zollinger and Ellison consisted of fulminating ulcer diathesis; recurrent ulceration despite intensive medical, radical surgical or radiation treatment, and the presence of a non-beta islet cell tumor of the pancreas. Neoplasms or hyperplasia of other endocrine organs, especially of the parathyroids, the pituitary and the adrenals, are present in 20% of patients with the Zollinger-Ellison syndrome.

A fulminating ulcer diathesis is present in about 90% of these patients and is associated with severe diarrhea in about half of these. The gastric hypersecretion is of remarkable proportion. In most instances, the 12-hour nocturnal secretion exceeds 2 liters with a free hydrochloric acid content of 100–300 mEq. (The normal volume is 400 ml with an acid output of 18 mEq.) Stimulation with histamine or insulin does not increase the acid production further.

Although the large volume of hydrochloric acid was assumed to cause the diarrhea, the latter may be present with or without gastric hypersecretion. The diarrhea may be sufficiently severe to cause death because of excessive loss of potassium. Frequently, the diagnosis of Zollinger-Ellison syndrome is not suspected until ulcer recurs shortly after standard operations for ulcer disease. Roentgenographically demonstrated multiple or unusually situated ulcers, as in the proximal jejunum or distal duodenum, may be the first clue to the presence of the Zollinger-Ellison syndrome.

ROENTGEN CHANGES.—The relative roentgenographic inaccessibility of the pancreas and the small size of islet cell tumors seldom permit demonstration by routine roentgen means. Barium examination is of little value in the diagnosis of insulin-producing tumors. An exception is the occasional tumor fortuitously situated adjacent to a portion of the distal antrum or duodenal loop.

The roentgen findings in the presence of the non-beta cell tumors of the Zollinger-Ellison syndrome reflect the physiologic changes caused by the tumor rather than the anatomic presence of the tumor itself. Persistent duodenal ulcers associated with giant mucosal folds in the stomach, marked retention of gastric secretions and hypermotility of the small intestine should suggest the diagnosis. Ulceration in unusual sites is also suggestive of the Zollinger-Ellison syndrome. Although 65% of the ulcers reported in the literature were located in the first part of the duodenum, 25% were found just distal to the ligament of Treitz. The remainder were in the second and third portions of the duodenum, the stomach and the distal esophagus. The duodenal sweep may appear to be dilated and atonic. Flocculation of barium in the duodenum and proximal jejunum is noted frequently. The contrast material within the small bowel is often diluted by the excessive secretions.

Selective arteriography of the celiac and superior mesenteric arteries may demonstrate an intensely vascular blush in instances of insulin-secreting islet cell tumors (Fig. 57, *D*). Madsen[4] performed such arteriography in 3 patients whose clinical and laboratory studies indicated hyperinsulinism. In each instance, a tumor stain was demonstrated that permitted preoperative localization of the tumor. In one patient with the Zollinger-Ellison syndrome, Ludin *et al.*[5] demonstrated a vascular blush in both a primary islet cell carcinoma and its hepatic metastasis.

PANCREATIC CYSTADENOMA

Benign cystadenomas comprise less than 10% of all cystic lesions of the pancreas. Among 23,551 surgical specimens at the Presbyterian Hospital, New York, Frantz[6] found 10 cystadenomas. Their presence during the ages from infancy to the eighth decade have been recorded, but they are most frequent in the middle-aged. The tumor predominates in females, in a ratio of about 9:1.

PATHOLOGIC CHANGES.—These tumors are thought to arise as cystic neoplasms from the pancreatic duct. Also suggested as etiologic possibilities are neoplastic proliferation of the pancreatic acinar epithelium and proliferation of displaced embryonic cells. Grossly, the cystadenoma presents a coarsely lobulated surface. Although it is well encapsulated, it may adhere to surrounding structures. The tumor may be situated in any portion of the pancreas, but is more common in the body or tail than in the head. Usually, the tumors are solitary and vary in diameter from 5 to 15 cm. The largest tumor in the series of Piper *et al.*[7] measured $25 \times 20 \times 20$ cm and the smallest 2.5 cm in diameter. Most often, the tumors consist of cystic cavities separated by connective tissue septa. The cystadenoma is usually a highly vascular tumor with numerous dilated veins commonly coursing over its

[4] Madsen, B.: Demonstration of pancreatic insulomas by angiography, Brit. J. Radiol. 39:488, July, 1966.

[5] Ludin, H., *et al.*: Failure to diagnose Zollinger-Ellison syndrome by pancreatic arteriography, Brit. J. Radiol. 39:494, July, 1966.

[6] *Op. cit.*

[7] Piper, C. E., *et al.*: Pancreatic cystadenomata: Report of 20 cases, J.A.M.A. 180:648, May 26, 1962.

capsule. The malignant counterpart of the cystadenoma, the cystadenocarci-noma, may invade the extrapancreatic tissues and adjacent structures.

CLINICAL FINDINGS.—The tumors are generally slow growing and often cause no symptoms. Of the 20 patients reported on by Piper *et al.,* 15 had a palpable abdominal mass. Jaundice is rare because of the infrequency of cystadenoma in the head of the pancreas. Diabetes may be associated with a very large lesion.

Symptoms, if present, may include upper abdominal pain, frequently aggravated by bending over. Anorexia, vomiting, abdominal distention and constipation may result from pressure on the neighboring stomach and colon.

ROENTGEN CHANGES.—Calcium was present in 2 of the 20 patients of Piper *et al.* They described the calcifications associated with cystadenoma as varying from a few small irregular particles to large calcifications of a sunburst pattern. Displacement of the barium-filled gastrointestinal tract, indistinguishable from that produced by other cysts and tumors of the pancreas, has been the most frequently recorded roentgen finding. Marked vascularity of the tumor bed has been observed repeatedly, and frequently a highly vascular mass demonstrated by arteriography may suggest the diag-nosis (Fig. 53).

PSEUDOCYSTS OF THE PANCREAS

Pseudocysts are by far the most common cystic lesions of the pancreas. Because of its location over the vertebral column, the pancreas is particu-larly vulnerable to blunt trauma. Howard and Jordan[8] estimated that 1–2% of abdominal wounds involve injury to the pancreas and that formation of pseudocysts complicates 15% of such injuries. Some authors have re-ported a traumatic etiology of pancreatic pseudocysts in as high as 20–50%. In a review of 35 reported cases of pancreatic pseudocysts in children, Shockman and Marasco[9] noted a traumatic etiology in 50%. In adults, how-ever, interstitial or hemorrhagic pancreatitis is the most frequent cause of pseudocyst formation. Berk and Haubrich[10] found pseudocysts in 23 of 197 patients hospitalized because of pancreatitis, an incidence of 2.9%. Since pancreatitis is the most common cause of pancreatic pseudocysts, they are most often present in the fourth and fifth decades of life.

PATHOLOGIC CHANGES.—Pancreatic pseudocysts are collections of fluid

[8] Howard. J. M., and Jordan, G. L.: *Surgical Disease of the Pancreas* (Philadelphia: J. B. Lippincott Company, 1960).

[9] Shockman, A. T., and Marasco, J. A.: Pseudocysts of the pancreas, Am. J. Roentgenol. 101:628, November, 1967.

[10] Berk, E. J., and Haubrich, W. S.: Cysts of the Pancreas, in Bockus, H. (ed.): *Gastroenterology* (2nd ed.; Philadelphia: W. B. Saunders Company, 1965), Vol. 3.

arising as a result of escape of trypsinogen and lipase from the pancreatic acini. Concurrent autolysis with destruction of the parenchyma is progressive. The activated enzymes are most commonly released into the lesser omental sac after rupture through the anterior wall of the pancreas. Severe chemical peritonitis results, the peritoneal and serosal surfaces producing profuse inflammatory exudate. Loculation of the inflammatory process results in a pseudocyst. The cyst may be situated within the pancreatic substance but more often is adjacent to the pancreas. No significant predilection has been noted in the head or in the body or tail of the pancreas. Most pseudocysts are situated in the region of the lesser peritoneal sac. The cyst may extend anteriorly into the greater omentum or into the mesocolon.

Pseudocysts are relatively large, their volumes ranging from 100 ml to several liters.

CLINICAL FINDINGS.—A history of previous pancreatitis or trauma precedes the discovery of a pancreatic pseudocyst in most instances. The pseudocyst may form after the initial episode of pancreatitis but is more likely to arise in the course of recurring or relapsing pancreatitis. Post-traumatic pseudocysts may be the result of either blunt or penetrating abdominal trauma.

Pain is the most frequent symptom of pancreatic pseudocyst. Most of the patients complain of diffuse pain across the midepigastrium, frequently referred to the hypochondrium, more often to the left than to the right. Nausea, vomiting, fever, diarrhea and hydrothorax may also be observed. An epigastric mass is a usual physical finding in the patient with pseudocyst, in contrast to the infrequent palpation of a mass in patients with pancreatic neoplasms. The explanation for this difference lies in the frequency with which the pseudocysts extend anteriorly into the greater omentum or mesocolon. Of 21 patients with pancreatic pseudocysts reviewed by Shockman and Marasco, all but 1 were chronic alcoholics. Glycosuria or hyperglycemia, or both, are present in 50% of the patients, and in 40% the serum amylase levels are elevated.

ROENTGEN CHANGES.—Pancreatic lithiasis may be revealed in patients with pseudocysts of inflammatory origin. The barium-filled stomach, duodenum, jejunum or colon may be displaced by a pseudocyst of sufficient size (Fig. 55). There is no roentgen evidence of direct invasion of the displaced structures; however, differentiation from carcinoma of the pancreas is usually not possible.

Although arteriography may demonstrate displacement and stenosis of adjacent vascular structures, differentiation from pancreatic carcinoma has not been reliable.

Other types of cysts of the pancreas include retention, congenital and parasitic cysts. Congenital cysts are believed to result from anomalous development of the pancreatic ducts. The manner of this development is analogous to that postulated for the origin of congenital cysts of the kidney and liver. The cysts range in size from microscopic lesions to diameters of 3–5 cm.

Retention cysts are believed to result from obstruction of one of the major pancreatic ducts. They have been described in association with pancreatic lithiasis, chronic pancreatitis and trauma. This type of cyst is usually smaller than the congenital type. Retention cysts are usually multiple, their diameters rarely exceeding several centimeters, and they are of little clinical significance.

Seldom seen in the United States are two other types of cysts. These are the cysts caused by parasites, as a direct result of infestation, as in hydatid disease, and those secondary to duct obstruction, as by Ascaris.

The roentgenographic manifestations of these cystic lesions, as with all pancreatic masses, vary with the location, size and direction of growth. If the cysts are large enough to affect adjacent structures, their appearance on roentgenograms is nonspecific, and a precise diagnosis is seldom possible.

Figure 44.—Carcinoma of the head of the pancreas.

A, upper gastrointestinal series. A faint impression is noted along the inner aspect of the descending duodenum (**a**). The duodenal mucosa has a somewhat spiked appearance. These roentgenographic changes are of minimal degree and are nonspecific. Swelling of the head of the pancreas, as in acute pancreatitis, may give an identical appearance.

B, upper gastrointestinal series. The roentgen changes involving the duodenal sweep are more pronounced than in *A*. Two smooth, nodular impressions (**arrows**) are present along the upper margins of the third portion of the duodenum. The mucosa is not distorted or destroyed. The postbulbar portion of the duodenum (**a**) is moderately narrow, the result of compression by tumor or by a dilated common duct. Such narrowing must be observed as constant on fluoroscopic examination, since duodenal spasm may show identical changes, particularly in instances of postbulbar ulcer.

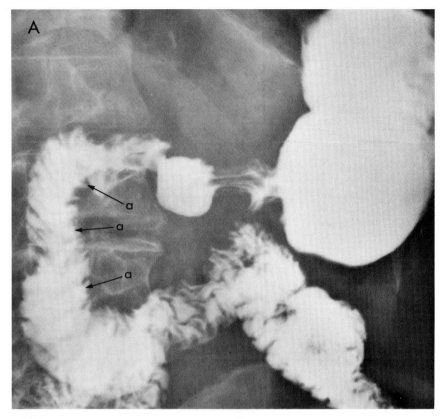

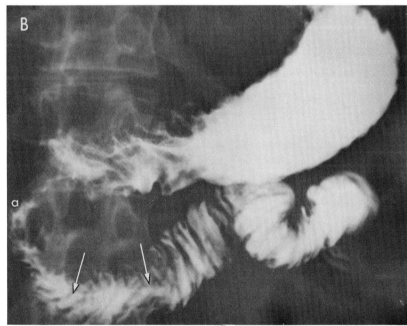

Figure 44 · Carcinoma of the Head / 127

Figure 45.—Carcinoma of the pancreas.

A, upper gastrointestinal series, demonstrating mucosal effacement of the gastric antrum (**a**), descending duodenum (**b**) and the third portion of the duodenum (**c**) by a mass in the head of the pancreas. Diagnosis was carcinoma of the head of the pancreas.

B (same patient as in A), T-tube cholangiogram, showing the common bile duct (**d**) narrowed distally by an extrinsic mass. There is, however, egress into the duodenum (**b**).

C, upper gastrointestinal series, lateral view. A retrogastric mass causes a localized impression on the body of the stomach (**arrows**). Diagnosis was carcinoma of the body and tail of the pancreas.

D, upper gastrointestinal series, right anterior oblique view. The lesser curvature of the stomach is rigid and straightened (**arrows**). In addition, barium fills an irregular ulcer (**e**) of the lesser curvature. Diagnosis was carcinoma of the body and tail of the pancreas, with invasion and ulceration of the stomach.

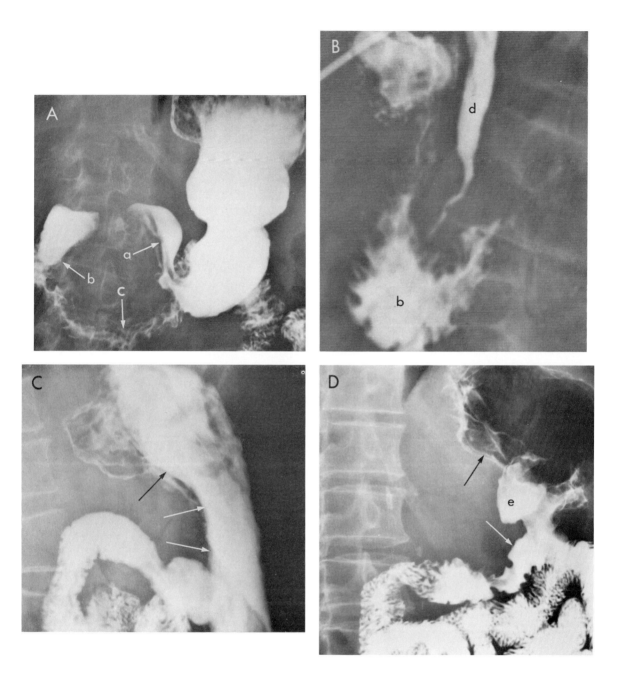

Figure 45 · Carcinoma / 129

Figure 46.—Carcinoma of the pancreas.

A, upper gastrointestinal series. An annular constricting lesion (**arrows**) involves the descending duodenum. This appearance is relatively specific for malignancy throughout the gastrointestinal tract. This was a carcinoma of the head of the pancreas.

B, upper gastrointestinal series. A large mass has caused a smooth impression along the entire lesser curvature of the stomach (**arrows**). Diagnosis was carcinoma of the body of the pancreas.

C, barium enema examination. The gallbladder (**a**) is opacified by incidental oral cholecystography. A calcified mass is present slightly below and medial to the gallbladder (**b**). This was a calcified carcinoma of the head of the pancreas.

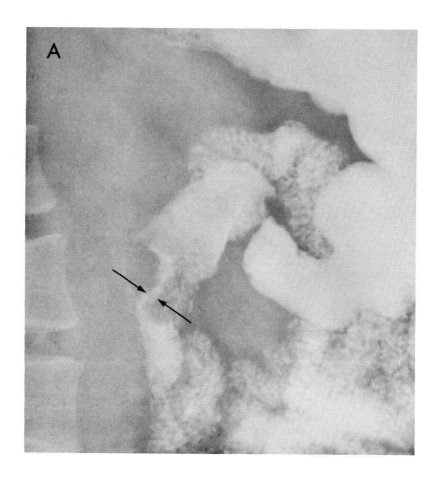

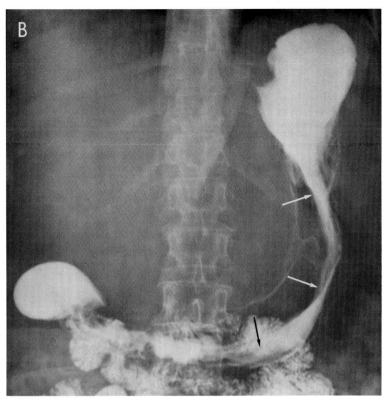

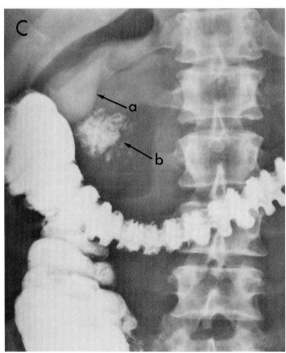

Figure 46 · Carcinoma / 131

Figure 47.—Zollinger-Ellison syndrome.

This patient complained of gastric hyperacidity and recurring gastric and duodenal ulcers. Marked nonopaque gastric residue was repeatedly observed flouroscopically.

This prone roentgenogram of the upper intestinal tract reveals evidence of an active postbulbar ulcer (**arrow**). Note the distended, fluid-filled jejunal loops indicative of gastric hypersecretion.

At operation, a non-insulin-producing (non-beta) islet cell tumor of the pancreas was found.

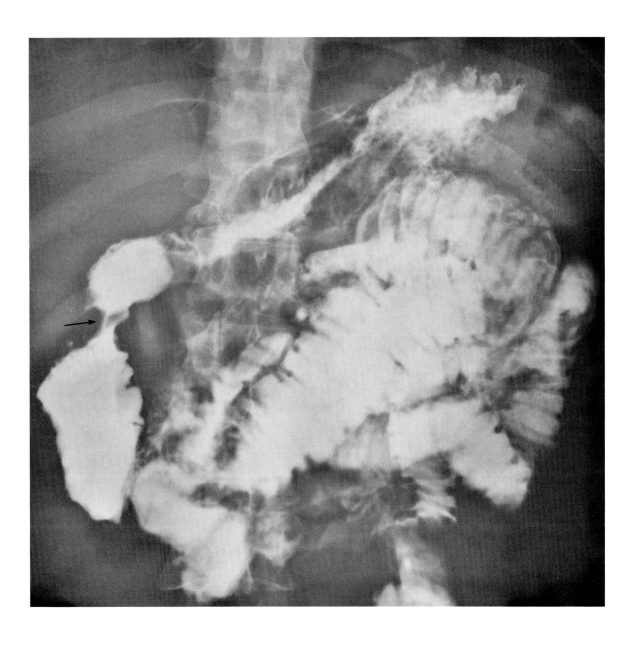

Figure 47 · Zollinger-Ellison Syndrome / 133

Figure 48.—Zollinger-Ellison syndrome.

Prone posteroanterior barium study: Revealing evidence of gastric hyper-secretion, manifested by the presence of a considerable nonopaque residue which has diluted and flocculated the barium. The second and third portions of the duodenum revealed pronounced hyperirritability, but no ulcers were demonstrated roentgenographically or surgically.

(*Continued* in Figure 49.)

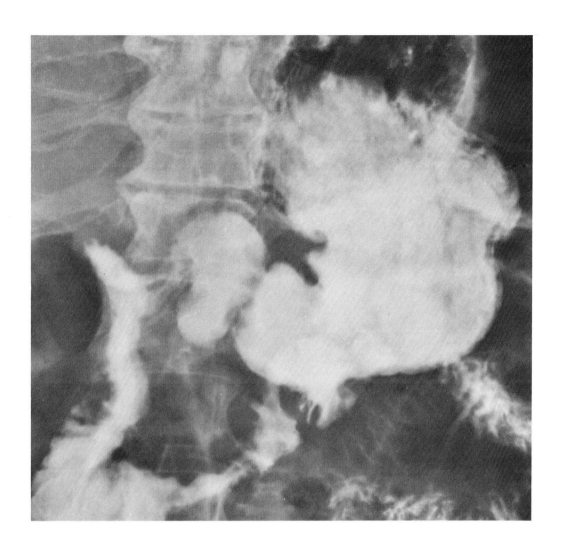

Figure 48 · Zollinger-Ellison Syndrome / 135

Figure 49.—Zollinger-Ellison syndrome (same patient as in Figure 48).

A, early arterial phase of celiac artery arteriogram: The tumor blush in the tail of the pancreas is obvious (**arrows**).

B, late arterial phase of same arteriogram: The tumor blush is seen to better advantage (**arrows**).

The patient had complained of steatorrhea. A benign non-insulin-producing (non-beta) islet cell tumor was removed from the tail of the pancreas.

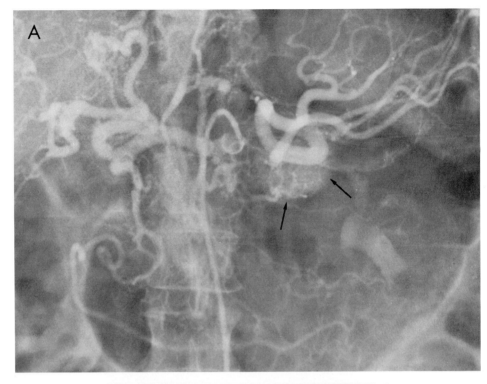

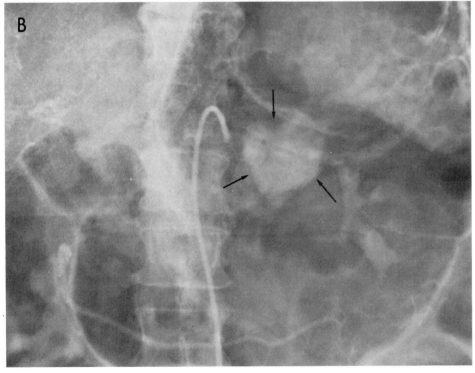

Figure 49 · Zollinger-Ellison Syndrome / 137

Figure 50.—Zollinger-Ellison syndrome.

This patient had had a papillary and follicular carcinoma of the thyroid which was treated surgically and cured. Four years later, recurring gastric and duodenal ulcers appeared which did not respond to medical management. She eventually died of a massive intestinal hemorrhage. At autopsy, the pancreas was displaced by a 1,000-Gm nodular mass which proved to be a non-insulin-producing (non-beta) islet cell carcinoma. Metastases were found in the stomach and duodenum.

A, oblique gastrointestinal exposure: Demonstrating pronounced anterior displacement of the stomach (**arrows**) by the pancreatic mass.

B, splenoportogram: Revealing striking cut-off (**arrow**) of portal circulation by extrinsic pressure or invasion by pancreatic tumor.

(*Continued* in Figure 51.)

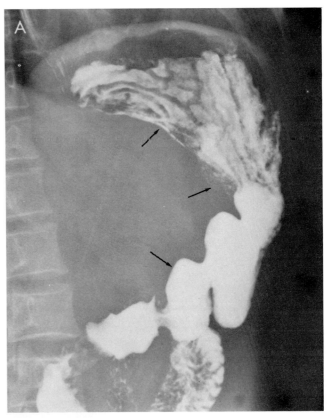

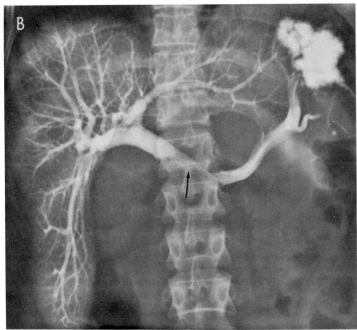

Figure 50 · Zollinger-Ellison Syndrome / 139

Figure 51.—Zollinger-Ellison syndrome (same patient as in Figure 50).

A, early phase of arteriogram: Showing the common hepatic artery (**a**) displaced upward. **Arrows** point to irregularities and scalloping along its inferior margin due to tumor pressure. **b,** splenic artery; **c,** superior mesenteric artery; **d,** inferior pancreaticoduodenal artery; **e,** gastroduodenal artery; **f,** vessels feeding the metastatic nodule in the liver.

B, late arterial phase: Revealing to better advantage the extensive pancreatic tumor (**arrows**). Note the clarity with which the metastatic lesion in the liver is now demonstrated (**x**).

Figures 50 and 51, courtesy of Dr. Gerald D. Dodd, Houston, Tex.

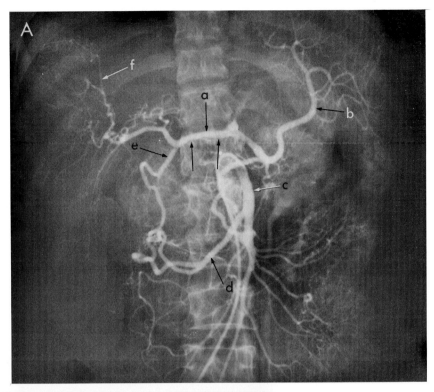

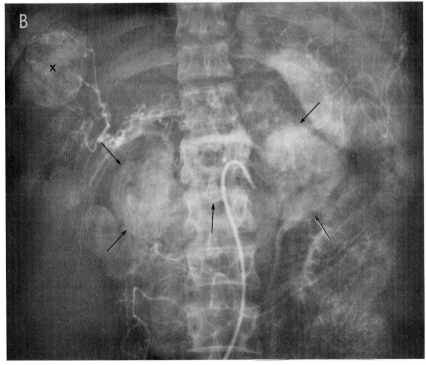

Figure 51 · Zollinger-Ellison Syndrome / 141

Figure 52.—Reticulum cell sarcoma of the pancreas.

A, anteroposterior 5-minute intravenous urogram, showing a normal right kidney but failing to demonstrate the left kidney. The carbon dioxide-filled stomach is displaced to the right by a mass, seemingly in the left upper quadrant.

B, anteroposterior 2-hour intravenous urogram, demonstrating the left kidney (for the first time in the series) with rather pronounced caliectasis but no evidence of the renal pelvis. It was believed that either there was a mass in the renal hilus or a tumor anterior and medial to the kidney was producing extrinsic pressure on it.

C, anteroposterior 3-hour intravenous urogram made 30 minutes after a barium swallow, revealing a widened duodenal loop (**a**) and displacement of the left kidney (**b**). A suspicion that the pancreas was enlarged was confirmed at operation.

This 4-year-old patient was seen because of a huge abdominal mass and anemia.

Figure 52, courtesy of Hope, J. W., and Koop, C. E.: M. Radiog. & Photog., vol. 38, no. 1, 1962.

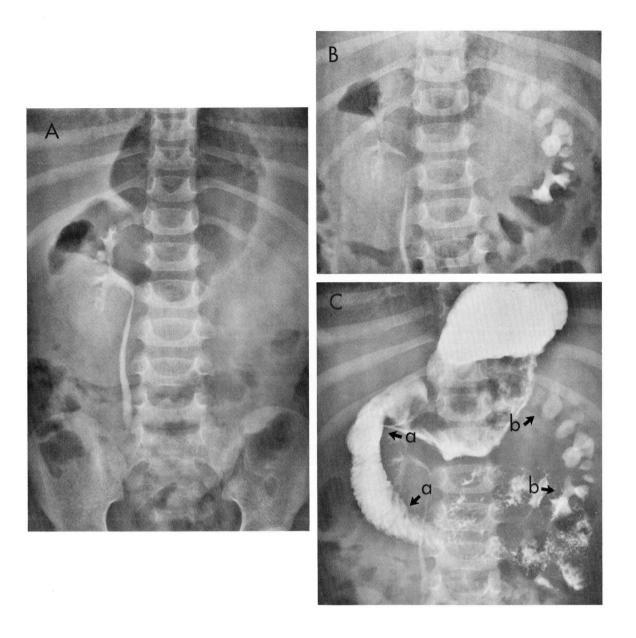

Figure 52 · Reticulum Cell Sarcoma / 143

Figure 53.—Pancreatic cystadenoma (all figures from same patient).

A, upper gastrointestinal series, with the patient prone. The duodenal sweep is widened and the duodenal mucosa effaced by a large mass in the head of the pancreas (**arrows**).

B, aortogram, arterial phase, with the patient prone. Large tumor vessels are seen in the region of the mass (**a**). The aorta is displaced to the left (**b**).

C, aortogram, late phase. An intense tumor blush is now apparent (**c**).

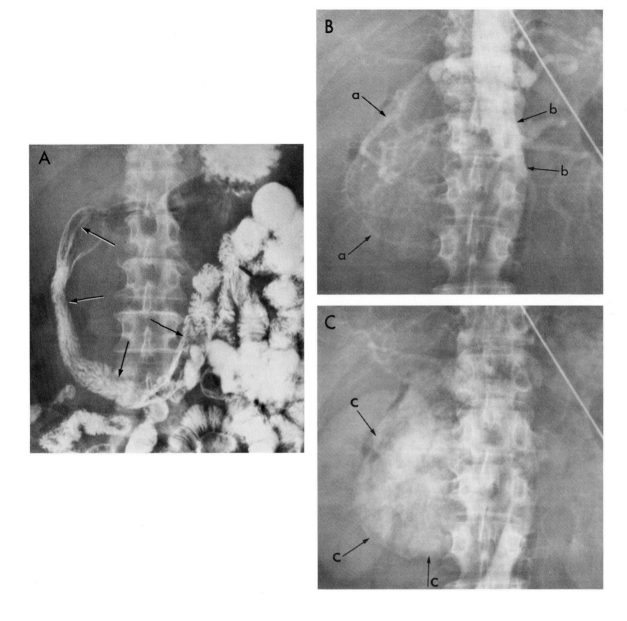

Figure 53 · Cystadenoma / 145

Figure 54.—Pancreatic pseudocyst.

Oral cholecystogram, revealing a huge mass (**arrows**) in the right mid-abdomen, displacing the gallbladder (**a**) to the left of the midline. This is an unusual manifestation of pancreatic pseudocyst.

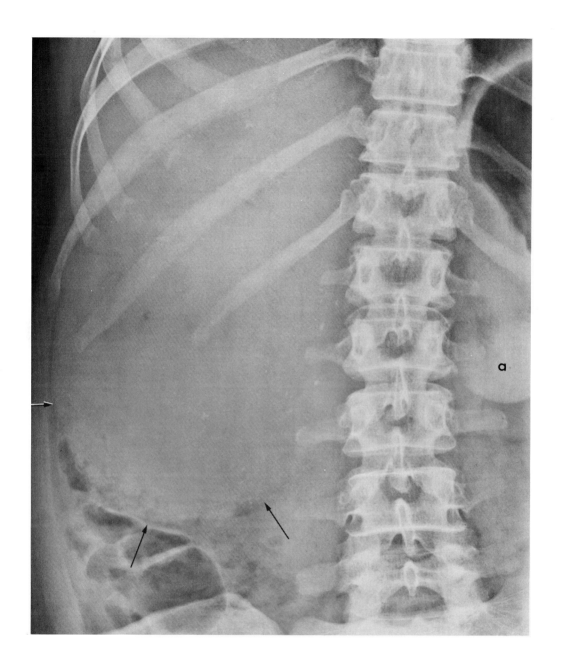

a

Figure 54 · Pseudocyst / 147

Figure 55.—Traumatic pseudocyst of the pancreas.

A, anteroposterior roentgenogram after barium swallow, made 11 days after a boy of 7 fell from his bicycle. The duodenal loop is widened (**a**), and there is evidence of extrinsic pressure from below (**b**) on the antral portion of the stomach, indicating a mass in the head of the pancreas.

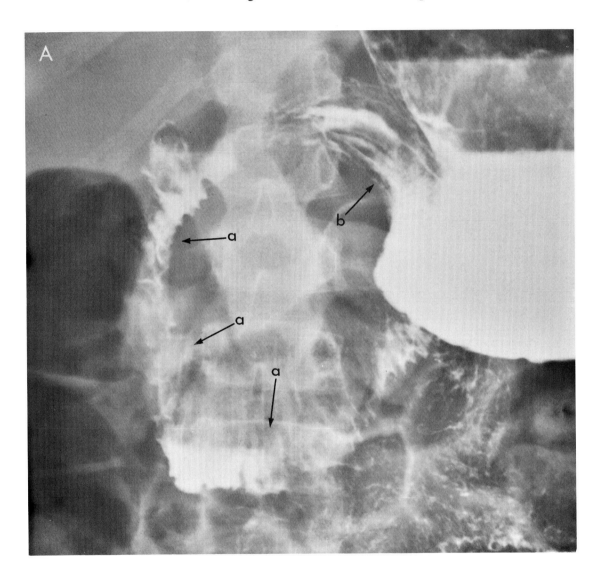

B, anteroposterior roentgenogram obtained 2 weeks after **A.** The duodenal loop is normal. The boy had remained asymptomatic for 4 years thereafter.

Figure 55, courtesy of Hope, J. W., and Koop, C. E.: M. Radiog. & Photog., vol. 38, no. 1, 1962.

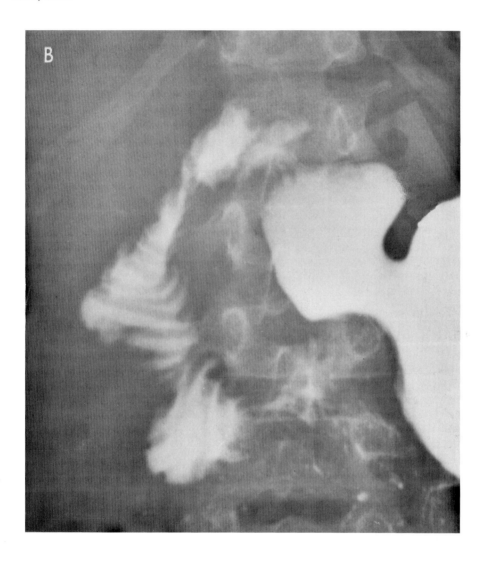

Figure 55 · Traumatic Pseudocyst / 149

Figure 56.—Ectopic Pancreas.

A, with the patient in prone position, a discrete, sharply defined filling defect is evident in the descending duodenum (**arrow**).

B, with another patient in right anterior oblique position, a filling defect is apparent within the antrum of the stomach (**arrows**). In the defect is a tiny collection of barium, contained in an atretic pancreatic duct.

C, with the patient in a somewhat more right anterior oblique position than in *B,* a sharply marginated mass is demonstrated in the gastric antrum (**arrows**) with a central fleck of barium within an atretic duct.

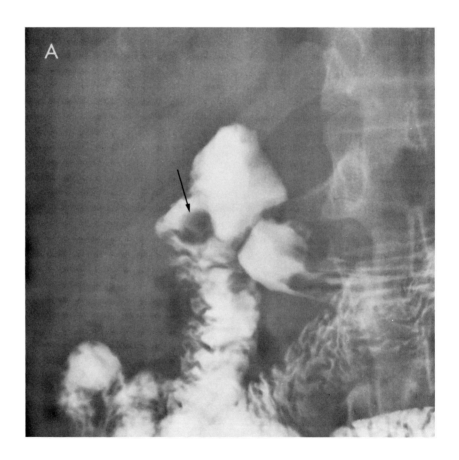

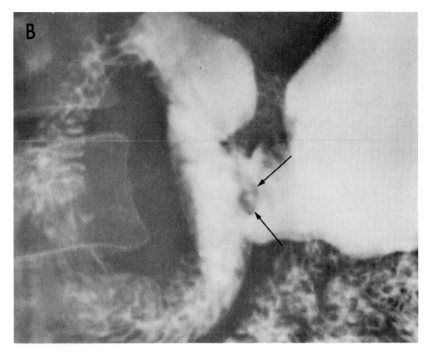

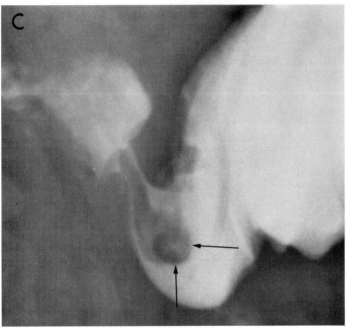

Figure 56 · Ectopic Pancreas / 151

Figure 57.—Special diagnostic methods.

A, percutaneous transhepatic cholangiogram, exposed with the patient supine. The common bile duct (**a**) is markedly dilated and is terminated abruptly by an intraluminal lesion, causing shelflike margins of the contrast material. This is the typical appearance of a common bile duct calculus.

B, percutaneous transhepatic cholangiogram, exposed with the patient supine. The common bile duct (**a**) and the cystic duct (**b**) are markedly dilated. The common bile duct is obstructed distally by a lesion that has caused tapered narrowing of the column of contrast material. This appearance is typical of an obstruction of the common bile duct by carcinoma of the head of the pancreas.

C, hypotonic duodenography. An opaque catheter has been introduced into the duodenum and barium injected. The atony of the duodenum permits excellent evaluation of the duodenal mucosa. The mucosa along the inner margin of the duodenum has a spiked appearance (**arrows**), secondary to mucosal infiltration or edema, or both. In addition, there is a faint, smooth impression on the mucosa at the junction of the second and third portions (**a**).

D, selective celiac and superior mesenteric arteriogram. The tip of the upper catheter is in the celiac artery, the lower catheter in the superior mesenteric artery. This relatively late phase of the arteriogram demonstrates a faint blush in the region of the head of the pancreas (**arrows**). At surgery, an insulinoma was found.

Figure 57, *C,* courtesy of Dr. Marcia K. Bilbao, Portland, Ore.

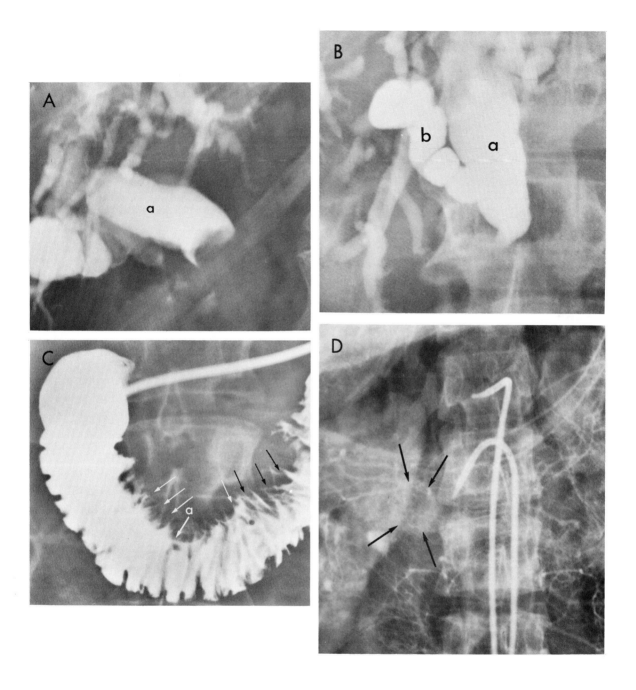

Figure 57 · Special Diagnostic Methods / 153

PART 5

The Adrenal Glands

Characteristics of Adrenal Neoplasms

NEOPLASMS OF THE adrenal glands may be secondary by direct extension of malignant lesions from adjacent organs, or through lymphatic, retrograde venous or arterial dissemination from distant sites. The initial site of the malignant neoplasm is usually the medulla, but the tumor may extend to involve the cortex. At necropsy, metastatic involvement of the adrenals may be present in more than 10% of cases and more often this is bilateral than unilateral. Usually the origin is from the lung, breast, stomach, colon, biliary system, and kidney. The smaller metastatic nodules are generally spherical and well defined. Several metastatic nodules of various sizes may be present in a single adrenal body. The tumors may attain great size and may extend directly beyond the adrenal.

The homologous tumors, which are the clinically important lesions and will be discussed at length, may or may not elaborate excessive quantities of hormones.

Certain tumors of the adrenal glands may arise from cells that are not limited to the adrenal glands, resulting in a fibroma, myoma, neurofibroma, lipoma, hemangioma, lymphangioma, melanoma or fibrosarcoma, but these are rare.

TUMOR-LIKE LESIONS

CYSTS

Most cysts that occur in the adrenal glands either are pseudocysts resulting from cystic degeneration of hematomas or adenomas or are dilated angiomatous cavities. These cavities are more frequent in the lymphangiomas, where they are often multilocular. True glandular cysts and parasitic (echinococcus) cysts have been described. The cysts are more common in females than in males. The diameter of the cysts may be as large as 30 cm. They occur equally on both sides. The fibrous wall of about 35% of all cysts contains calcium which, in most instances, is not visible on plain films but may be demonstrated by special techniques (Fig. 58).

CORTICAL NODULES

These nodules are spherical, usually encapsulated masses of cells in the cortex, capsule or periadrenal fat. The cells are similar to those of the adrenal cortex. They are usually bilateral and their diameters range from less than 1 mm to 4 cm. Often they are multiple and are observed in about one third of autopsies. When large, roentgenographic differentiation from a cortical adenoma may be difficult.

MYELOLIPOMAS

Myelolipomas are masses of fatty tissue in the medulla or cortex that contain cells like those of bone marrow. The usually solitary mass measures a few millimeters to 6 cm in diameter. Calcification is rare. Such masses are of no clinical significance but, when appearing large on roentgenograms, may resemble clinically significant masses.

ADRENAL CORTEX TUMORS

CORTICAL ADENOMAS

These benign, encapsulated, round, smooth neoplasms are usually single and may become extremely large (Fig. 59). Hemorrhage, necrosis and degenerative cyst formation occur in the tumor. The cells that compose an adenoma vary and often lack uniformity, are pleomorphic and sometimes contain giant cells. Their arrangement may be irregular, and they may be clustered or columnar.

Adenomas associated with primary hyperaldosteronism are usually small, varying from 1 to 5 cm in diameter. They are composed mainly of large lipid-laden cells. Nonfunctioning adenomas may be composed of cells of similar appearance.

CARCINOMA

Carcinoma of the adrenal cortex is relatively uncommon and is usually associated with endocrine dysfunction. The tumor tends to be larger than an adenoma (Figs. 68 and 69). Some functioning carcinomas, however, may be small. The circulation of the tumor may be abundant, causing hemorrhage or necrosis. The cells of some tumors appear to be typical of malignancy, but, cytologically, others are similar to adenomas. In such instances, the true nature of the tumor may be indicated by invasion into the capsule or by metastasis. Adrenal carcinoma may spread by direct growth into the adrenal veins and the inferior vena cava. Metastatic growth is mainly to para-aortic lymph nodes, lungs and liver.

Adrenal cortical tumors arising in adrenal rests may be situated in the male anywhere from the testicle to the kidney and in the female from the ovary to the kidney. These tumors may or may not produce hormonal changes.

HYPERPLASIA

Hyperplasia of the adrenal cortex is bilateral and may be nodular or diffuse. *Nodular hyperplasia,* which is more frequent, is usually of no clinical significance and the glands are of normal size or slightly enlarged. This condition is described earlier, under cortical nodules.

Diffuse hyperplasia is infrequent and is usually associated with clinical endocrine abnormality. As a rule, both glands are enlarged. The hyperplasia involves the cells of the zona reticulata which, in adrenal hyperplasia of the congenital virilizing syndrome, may replace most of the fascicular zone or may comprise almost the entire cortex. In Cushing's syndrome, the zona reticulata is increased in width, but frequently the zona fasciculata is equally prominent.[1]

The clinical features of the adrenal cortical neoplasms to be discussed below are outlined in Table 1.[2]

TABLE 1.—CLINICAL FEATURES OF ADRENAL CORTICAL NEOPLASMS

1. Nonhormonal tumors. Symptoms are the result of mechanical pressure or infiltration of a nonfunctioning tumor.
2. Cushing's syndrome. Main symptoms are the result of excessive secretion of cortisol.
   a. Bilateral adrenal hyperplasia.
   b. Unilateral adrenal adenoma or carcinoma (often virilization).
3. Adrenogenital syndrome. Main symptoms result from excessive secretion of androgens.
   a. Congenital adrenal hyperplasia (defect of cortisol synthesis).
   b. Virilizing unilateral adrenal tumors.
4. Primary hyperaldosteronism. Symptoms are caused by excessive secretion of aldosterone.
   a. Aldosterone-producing tumor.
   b. Adrenal hyperplasia.
5. Feminizing syndrome. Symptoms are due to excessive secretion of estrogens often accompanied with virilization. Adrenal tumor usually malignant.

---

[1] Karsner, H. T.: Tumors of the Adrenal, in *Atlas of Tumor Pathology,* Sect. VIII, fasc. 29 (Washington, D.C.: Armed Forces Institute of Pathology, 1950); Anderson, W. A. D.: *Pathology* (5th ed.; St. Louis: C. V. Mosby Company, 1966); Wilkins, L.: *The Diagnosis and Treatment of Endocrine Disorders in Childhood and Adolescence* (3rd ed.; Springfield, Ill.: Charles C Thomas, Publisher, 1965).

[2] Williams, R. H.: *Textbook of Endocrinology* (4th ed.; Philadelphia: W. B. Saunders Company, 1962); Meyers, M. A.: *Diseases of the Adrenal Glands: Radiologic Diagnosis* (Springfield, Ill.: Charles C Thomas, Publisher, 1963); Steinbach, H. L., *et al.*: Diagnosis of adrenal neoplasms by contrast media, Radiology 69:664, November, 1957.

Characteristics of Adrenal Neoplasms / 159

NONHORMONAL TUMORS

Asymptomatic cortical tumors are common, are usually benign and are found incidentally. The symptom-producing tumors, usually occurring in adults, are generally malignant. They are more common on the left side than on the right, but may develop in aberrant adrenals. The symptoms are similar to those produced by other retroperitoneal tumors and depend on the size of the tumor and infiltration of adjacent tissues. Metastasis frequently spreads to liver, lungs, retroperitoneal lymph nodes and kidneys.

CUSHING'S SYNDROME

This is a relatively rare disease that is about four times as common in females as in males. It may be noted in childhood, but generally occurs in the third and fourth decades. The syndrome may result from a hyperfunction of the pituitary gland or hypothalamus, leading to excessive secretion of cortisol, which produces most of the systemic manifestations. Rarely, a basophil adenoma of the pituitary, which does not cause sellar enlargement, or occasionally a chromophobe adenoma of the pituitary, which may or may not increase sellar size, secretes ACTH, causing adrenal hyperplasia. Primary adrenal cortical hyperplasia, independent of ACTH secretion and therefore autonomous, is less common. The hyperplastic adrenals may be large or of normal size. In about 15% of the patients, the syndrome is produced by an adenoma or carcinoma of the adrenal cortex. These tumors are usually autonomous, but some have been shown to be dependent on ACTH secretion. Hyperplasia and Cushing's syndrome may be associated with non-endocrine tumors, such as oat cell carcinoma of the lung, neoplasms of the thymus, islet cells, colon, thyroid, ovary and gallbladder and arrhenoblastoma.

The hyperplastic glands, adenomas and carcinomas secrete excess cortisol, leading to the predominant features of Cushing's syndrome. Pituitary-dependent hyperplasia, adenomas and particularly carcinomas secrete additional androgenic hormones that produce virilization.

The symptoms and signs of Cushing's syndrome include: obesity, accentuated on the trunk and face and sparing the extremities; weakness; thin skin with bruisability, striae, and acne; hypertrichosis in females; diminished sexual function and amenorrhea; psychic changes; hypertension; osteoporosis, often with fractures; renal calculi; hirsutism, and virilism.

The positive results of laboratory studies include increased urinary excretion of 17-hydroxycorticoids and 17-ketogenic steroids. Excretion levels are usually further increased three to five times over the control values by stimulation with ACTH (not in adrenal carcinoma). Dexamethasone suppresses the excretion levels. Values fall to at least one half the basal levels in normal patients and in those with hyperplasia, but not in those with adenoma or carcinoma. The glucose tolerance test indicates a diabetic tendency. Polycythemia and elevated hemoglobin are characteristic. Eosinophils and lymphocytes are usually diminished.

ROENTGEN EXAMINATION.—*Plain roentgenograms and tomography.*— At times, the normal adrenal gland may be visible on plain roentgenograms as a triangular shadow surrounded by fat and situated adjacent to the upper pole of the kidneys. In some instances, tomograms may be necessary to obliterate confusing shadows that tend to obscure the adrenals. A normal size and shape of the adrenals would exclude a tumor but not hyperplasia, since in many instances hyperplastic glands are of normal size. Sufficiently large tumors may be identified on plain roentgenograms and to better advantage on tomograms. Calcification in adrenal tumors is uncommon but, when present, may aid in identification of the lesion. It may be present in small spherical foci or may be irregular and occurs in either benign or malignant tumors (Figs. 66, *C;* 67, *B;* 70, *B*). Calcification of the adrenals has been described in adrenal cysts (Fig. 58), Addison's disease, Niemann-Pick disease, familial cholesterosis, neuroblastoma (Fig. 79, *A*) and pheochromocytoma (Fig. 82, *C*).

Large adrenal masses displace the kidney caudally and occasionally cranially and cause rotation along its longitudinal axis. These changes may be seen on plain roentgenograms or, more frequently, on urograms (Figs. 63, *B;* 66, *B;* 67, *A;* 69, *A;* 70, *B;* 87, *A*). Displacement of adjacent viscera, such as the stomach, duodenum and colon, may be seen on barium examination (Fig. 69, *C* and *D*). Malignant tumors may infiltrate organs or tissues.

Extraperitoneal pneumography.—Gas introduced into tthe extraperitoneal tissues passes along the tissue planes, outlining the psoas shadows and retroperitoneal space. Some of the gas passes inside Gerota's fascia that surrounds the kidney and adrenal. The adrenal gland is attached to the apex of Gerota's fascia and does not descend significantly when the patient assumes the erect position. The kidney is more mobile, and thus the erect position may separate these two structures, permitting easier identification. On rare occasions, this examination may lead to pulmonary gas embolism, particularly if insoluble gas such as room air is used. We prefer to use oxygen, which is more soluble and which, in our hands, has caused no serious complications, although several deaths have been reported elsewhere. Carbon dioxide is more soluble and more readily absorbed but is more

Characteristics of Adrenal Neoplasms / 161

difficult to use. With oxygen, the roentgenograms may be repeated at later intervals, allowing better distribution of gas (Fig. 64).

Hyperplastic adrenals may appear to be of normal size and shape, or they may be enlarged, with a convex rather than the usual concave border. Frequently, extensive fatty areolar tissue surrounds these adrenals, preventing a sharp outline of gas. Benign neoplasms and encapsulated malignant tumors vary in size. The gland may be only slightly enlarged and its contours concave. Later, the angle of the triangle-shaped adrenal becomes rounded and the tumor assumes an oval shape (Fig. 66); when very large, it becomes spherical (Fig. 69). In Cushing's syndrome, the opposite adrenal is atrophic (Figs. 63, *A;* 66, *A*). Malignant tumors that spread into adjacent tissues may be poorly outlined. With extra-adrenal cortisol-producing tumors, both adrenals appear small.

Angiography.—Aortography, selective adrenal arteriography or retrograde adrenal venography may be applied to demonstrate the normal and abnormal adrenal glands (Figs. 59, *C*; 62, *B*; 65, *C* and *D*; and 67, *C*). Epinephrine injected into vessels a few seconds prior to the injection of contrast medium constricts the renal and most other visceral vessels but does not significantly affect the adrenal vessels. Relatively vascular hyperplastic adrenals and adrenal tumors are demonstrated by aortography. Their delineation may be improved, however, by selective arteriography of the inferior phrenic artery, the middle adrenal arteries and the renal arteries, which provide branches to the gland. The arteries supplying the tumor may appear to be normal, but more numerous and increased in caliber or abnormal in contour and distribution. Venography is done selectively through a catheter placed in the adrenal vein (Fig. 62).

SKELETAL ABNORMALITIES.—Diffuse osteoporosis of the skeleton is common with Cushing's syndrome. As with other forms of osteoporosis, spongy bone is more affected than compact cortical bone. Rarefied mottling of the skull, sometimes present, may disappear on treatment of Cushing's syndrome, but osteoporosis persists. Ischemic necrosis of the femoral and humeral heads develops as well as of other sites. The bones are brittle and fracture readily, sometimes associated with little pain. The final conversion of callus to bone is impeded and large masses of callus may persist around fracture sites. The fractures are incurred most often in the ribs and spine (Figs. 64, *B*; 72). Horizontal sclerotic bands just below the superior end-plates or above the inferior end-plates of compressed vertebrae appear much more commonly with the osteoporosis of Cushing's syndrome than with other forms (Fig. 72).

In children, the growth and, to a lesser extent, maturation of the skeleton are arrested. Unlike in adults, treatment of Cushing's syndrome results in healing of the osteoporosis by the formation of new bone over old, or replacement of bone.

The sella turcica of the skull may be large in some patients with adrenal hyperplasia. With adrenal adenoma or carcinoma in childhood, the sella may be unusually small.

ADRENOGENITAL SYNDROME

The adrenogenital syndrome may be the result of adrenal hyperplasia or of tumor.

Congenital virilizing adrenal hyperplasia.—This is the most common cause of virilism and is seen about four times as often in females as in males. It is much more frequent in childhood than is Cushing's syndrome. The disorder is the result of a deficiency of one or more of the hydroxylating enzymes involved in the synthesis of cortisol. The reduction of cortisol stimulates increased activity of the anterior pituitary gland, which produces an excess of corticotropin. The corticotropin in turn acts on the adrenals, producing hyperplasia and an increased synthesis of androgens. The abnormality starts in utero and results in various forms of pseudohermaphroditism of external, but not internal, genitals in females. The malformations range from enlargement of the clitoris to a penile urethra communicating with the bladder. A more common appearance is enlargement of the clitoris with fusion of the labioscrotal folds, leaving a single opening at the base of the phallus that communicates with both the bladder and the vagina. Males usually appear to be normal at birth, but virilization in both male and female children becomes progressively apparent, with rapid growth, muscular development and maturation. A further description of the malformation of the genitourinary tract is beyond the scope of this discussion.

Excretion of 17-ketosteroids is greatly increased because of abnormal production of androgens by the adrenal cortex. Pregnanetriol excretion is also increased. Approximately one third of these children lose excessive quantities of salt, and clinical signs of acute adrenal insufficiency develop. Medication with cortisol or cortisone arrests metabolic abnormalities but, of course, does not alter the anatomic malformations.

The weight of the adrenal glands increases to as much as three times the normal. This virilizing form of adrenal hyperplasia is inherited as a mendelian recessive. The parents are heterozygous and usually normal clinically.

One of the rarest of adrenogenital syndromes is a complete *deficiency of steroid hormone production,* including 17-ketosteroids and testicular and ovarian hormones. In this disease, cholesterol does not serve as a precursor for active steroid hormones, but accumulates in the adrenals, testes and ovaries. This defect can affect both sexes, female external genitalia developing in phenotypic males from absence of androgenic influence in utero.

Virilizing adrenal tumor.—Adrenal neoplasms that cause virilism are more common in older children and adults. They may be adenomas or carcinomas (Figs. 70 and 71). They are not active in utero and development of external sex organs is normal. In the male, differentiation from congenital hyperplasia may be difficult, as both syndromes lead to precocious virilization or macrogenitosomia praecox. Adult males have testicular atrophy, impotence and sterility resulting from depression of pituitary gonadotropins by androgens. Excretion of 17-ketosteroids is increased with hyperplasia or tumor, but with tumors it is not ACTH-dependent and therefore not depressed by cortisol, as is the case with hyperplasia.

Roentgen diagnosis.—Adrenal hyperplasia or tumor is diagnosed roentgenologically by the methods used for Cushing's syndrome. Generally, the disease is readily diagnosed clinically and extraperitoneal pneumography or angiography is not necessary. Plain roentgenograms of the abdomen or urograms may be sufficient.

Skeletal system.—Skeletal maturation of the young infant is usually retarded, particularly if the syndrome is of the salt-losing type. Subsequently, both growth and maturation of the skeleton are accelerated, with maturation much more advanced (Fig. 60). Because of the advanced maturation, the epiphyses fuse early and the initially large bone is ultimately small. The onset of menstruation in females and of puberty in males corresponds to the skeletal maturation rather than to the chronologic age. The dental age is usually not greatly advanced, although the jaws are increased in size. Markedly advanced tooth development has been reported, particularly in older children. With the bone growth and skeletal maturation, the muscle mass is correspondingly increased. The trunk is relatively long compared to the extremities. The heart may be small, as it is in Addison's disease. With the salt-losing form, pyloric and duodenal obstruction may be present and the amount of gas in the bowel reduced. The obstruction is caused by spasm of the pylorus and dehydration, easily alleviated by correcting the metabolic disorder. It may be confused with pyloric stenosis.

Since virilizing adrenal tumors usually occur at a later age, skeletal maturation is less affected than in adrenal hyperplasia.

Aldosteronism

Aldosteronism is usually the result of an adrenal cortical adenoma but may also be associated with adrenal carcinoma. Infrequently, particularly in young individuals, the adrenals are hyperplastic or normal in size. These patients may have symptoms in childhood, and the disease has been called congenital aldosteronism. Aldosterone causes retention of sodium and loss of potassium by the kidney. The symptoms of primary aldosteronism include muscular weakness, tetany, polyuria, polydipsia, hypertension and severe hypokalemic hypochloremic alkalosis. Excessive secretion of aldosterone is found in the adrenal veins by catheterization and in the urine.

ROENTGEN DIAGNOSIS.—Primary aldosteronism in four of five instances results from small adenomas, which usually weigh from 1 to 3 Gm. Because of their size, detection by roentgenographic methods is difficult. By extraperitoneal pneumography, we diagnosed two tumors, one weighing 8.4 Gm, the other 4.5 Gm, but in many cases establishment of the diagnosis has been unsuccessful. Aortography and selective arteriography with epinephrine also have been unrewarding in many patients. Adrenal venography often leads to intra-adrenal hemorrhage produced by rupture of the adrenal veins. Phlebography may be suggestive (Figs. 61 and 62). In some instances, surgical exploration of the adrenal glands is necessary.

FEMINIZING SYNDROME

This syndrome has been reported in several adult males in whom it caused testicular atrophy, gynecomastia and sometimes galactorrhea. The syndrome is rare in preadolescent boys but has been described in preadolescent girls, in whom it causes precocious development of breasts, vagina and uterus and secondary sex characteristics. Usually, the tumors in adult males are malignant and large and metastasize readily. Because of its large size, the tumor may be visible on plain roentgenograms of the abdomen or on intravenous urograms. Whether malignant or benign, the tumor may be calcified. The unusual small tumor may be diagnosed by extraperitoneal pneumography or angiography.

The feminization is produced by excessive secretion of estrogens. In most patients, urinary 17-ketosteroid values have also been increased. In children, the excess estrogen stimulates skeletal maturation and epiphyseal closure, but not growth.

ADRENAL MEDULLA TUMORS

Tumors of the medulla are composed of cells that are of immature or mature types. Those composed of the most immature types of cells (sympathicogonioma and neuroblastoma) are seen almost exclusively in early life and are highly malignant. Ganglioneuroma and pheochromocytoma, composed of the mature form, are benign, occurring mainly in adult life. Neuroblastomas in time may become transformed into ganglioneuromas.

NEUROBLASTOMA

Neuroblastoma (sympathicoblastoma) is one of the most common malignant neoplasms in infants and children and is limited almost exclusively to this age group. When it develops in adults, it is more often extra-adrenal.

The symptoms and signs of neuroblastoma depend on its size, extent of metastasis and the secondary effects of catecholamines secreted by the tumor or its metastasis.

The most common complaint is an abdominal mass, which often crosses the midline. Abdominal pain, fever, debility and bone pain may be present. If the neoplasm involves the chest, it may cause dyspnea, cough, tachypnea, wheezing, stridor or cyanosis. The liver and peripheral lymph nodes may be enlarged.

Neuroblastoma may arise from any site containing elements of the sympathetic nervous system. Almost half of them arise in the adrenal medulla. Others arise from ganglions in the cervical, thoracic, abdominal, celiac and pelvic regions and in the aortic bodies. Neuroblastoma also develops intracranially, in the nose and probably in the ganglions of the cranial nerves. Aberrant foci are situated in the skin and subcutaneous tissues, the kidney and the liver.

Microscopically, the tumor is extremely cellular, composed of small dark cells resembling lymphocytes whose characteristic feature is a circular grouping or rosette formation around a fine fibrillar network. It differs from sympathicogonioma in its greater maturity.

Local extension into lymphatics, adjacent tissues and viscera is common, and the tumor may become large. Metastasis may be widespread, even from a small primary tumor. The liver and skeletal system are frequent sites of metastatic growths. In infants younger than 1 year, the liver may be involved and enlarged massively. The lungs are usually spared until late in the disease. Neuroblastoma may regress spontaneously or may mature to ganglioneuroma, particularly in infants. In one of our patients, diffuse metastatic skeletal lesions were seen to change to ganglioneuromas; then, after many years, a lesion of the scapula resumed its malignant characteristics and resulted in death. Subcutaneous nodules are most common in young infants. At the time the tumor is discovered, and even when the primary lesion is small, it has already metastasized in most patients.

In some patients, the symptoms are the result of a high level of epinephrine and norepinephrine secreted by the tumor and its metabolite, vanillyl mandelic acid (VMA). The symptoms are hypertension, tachycardia, sweating, pallor and diarrhea. Even without these symptoms, the urinary metabolites, including catecholamines, dopamine and VMA, are usually increased, and their identification is of diagnostic importance as well as an aid in establishing the presence of residual or metastatic tumors.

ROENTGEN CHANGES.[3]—Plain roentgenograms reveal an abdominal mass in most instances (Figs. 73–75; 78, *A*; 79, *A*). The mass may extend beyond the midline and displace adjacent organs—the colon, stomach, kidney and ureter. Metastatic spread to the liver produces a large liver shadow, which may be the only abnormality. Calcification of the mass or of the regional lymph nodes is present in about one third of the patients (Figs. 73, *A*; 74; 78, *A* and *C*; 79, *A*). Usually, the calcification is finely stippled within the mass. In some tumors, the calcification may be confluent throughout its entirety. Calcification has been seen in metastatic neoplasms of the liver.

Urograms reveal displacement of the kidney in more than three fourths of the patients (Figs. 73, *B*; 74, *B*; 75, *B*). The displacement is usually downward and outward and the kidney is rotated. Tumors arising in the paravertebral ganglions displace the kidney laterally or upward, and the ureter laterally, depending on their positions. The tumor produces distortion of the calices and pelvis by compression, but only rarely does it cause the elongation and stretching of these structures that are seen with intrinsic renal lesions. Hydronephrosis from compression or invasion of the ureter or kidney pelvis is uncommon. Rarely, the kidney will not excrete the contrast material because of invasion of the renal vein or complete obstruction. Some of the pelvic neuroblastomas distort and displace the bladder and ureter (Fig. 76, *A*).

Intrathoracic neuroblastomas may be primary or secondary. Since the prognosis for primary intrathoracic lesions is far better than for extension from abdominal tumors, such extension from the abdomen should be ruled out. The primary tumor is usually in the posterior mediastinum, from the first to the twelfth vertebrae, and is almost always unilateral. The mass is lobulated or ill defined and often very large. Calcification is much less common than with intra-abdominal neuroblastomas, but gives the same roentgenographic appearance. The tumor may displace and narrow the adjacent ribs or invade the ribs and vertebrae. It may enlarge the intervertebral foramina.

Abdominal neuroblastomas may extend to widen the retroperitoneal and retropleural spaces in the thoracolumbar region and displace the medial

---

[3] Steinbach, H L., *et al.*: Retroperitoneal tumors in children, California Med. 78:263, April, 1953; Kincaid, O. W., *et al.*: Neuroblastoma: A roentgenologic and pathologic study, Am. J. Roentgenol. 78:420, September, 1957.

border of the lung. These changes indicate a spread of the tumor by contiguity or lymph node metastasis (Fig. 79, *A*).

Skeletal metastasis occurs in almost half of these patients, usually involving many bones. Unlike other metastatic neoplasms, those from neuroblastoma commonly invade the long bones distal to the elbow and knees. The lesions are generally at the ends of long bones, but often involve the entire bone. Lesions in the epiphyses are less common. The bones of the feet and hands are usually spared.

The lesions are predominantly lytic, but most often lytic and productive lesions are mixed (Figs. 78, *B*; 79, *B*). The flat bones of the pelvis, scapula and ribs in particular show evidence of bone proliferation. Destruction of the cortex is common in the long bones, and the tumor may be seen to extend into soft tissues. Periosteal bone proliferation is common in the long bones and skull, where it is usually in layers parallel to the cortex (Fig. 78, *B*). Occasionally, however, perpendicular spicules are present, particularly in the calvarium (Figs. 79 and 80). Often, multiple, small, irregular, indistinct lesions involve large areas of the skull (Fig. 80). Metastatic spread to the brain and meninges produces increased intracranial pressure and widened sutures. The skeletal margins of the sutures are also destroyed by metastatic tumor. The base of the skull, orbits, facial bones and mandible may be involved.

Bilateral symmetry is a characteristic feature of neuroblastomatous skeletal metastasis. It involves certain sites of the skeleton preferentially, such as the medial part of the proximal humeral metaphyses, which may be seen on roentgenograms of the chest, and the medial metaphyseal region of the distal ends of the femurs. Occasionally, a radiolucent stripe is present in the distal metaphysis, similar to that seen in leukemia.

GANGLIONEUROMA

Ganglioneuromas are found in both children and adults. About 50% occur in the abdomen, and about 25% of these are in the adrenal glands. These tumors secrete catecholamines, and there is increased excretion in the urine of norepinephrine, VMA, dopamine and homovanillic acid. These changes may lead to the same kind of diarrhea that may be confused with celiac disease and to hypertension.

Ganglioneuroma is a benign tumor composed of differentiated, large sympathetic ganglion cells and often of a few nerve fibers. It may occur from infancy to old age and often is an incidental finding at autopsy. It is less frequent in the adrenal gland than along the paravertebral sympathetic ganglions. The tumor is spherical or ovoid and sharply defined and is encapsulated. In or near the adrenal it is usually small but in other areas may be large. Morphologically similar tumors may metastasize, and others may present histologic evidence of malignancy.

ROENTGEN CHANGES.—Ganglioneuromas may appear as calcified or non-calcified masses, similar to the appearance of encapsulated neuroblastoma. The tumors grow slowly and may be large when detected. In the thorax, the lesions are round or oval in the paravertebral portion of the posterior mediastinum. Costal deformities consist of horizontal flattening, spreading of two adjacent ribs and irregularities of the margins.

PHEOCHROMOCYTOMA

Pheochromocytoma (chromaffinoma) arises at the site of chromaffin tissue, more commonly in the adrenal medulla and usually in young or middle-aged adults. In adults, about 10% of the tumors involve both adrenals and 10% are in extra-adrenal sites, usually near the kidneys, adrenals, aortic bodies or the organs of Zuckerkandl. They have been noted in the wall of the urinary bladder and appendix. Tumors arising from extra-adrenal chromaffin tissue are called paragangliomas.

Pheochromocytomas are usually less than 10 cm in diameter, are circumscribed and often contain cystic necrotic or hemorrhagic areas. Histologically, large irregular or polyhedral cells are present, with groups of cells surrounded by a stroma of vascular fine connective tissue. A predominant spindle cell pattern is seen in the rare malignant pheochromocytomas.

The symptoms and signs of these tumors may consist of pallor, sweating, headache, anxiety, convulsions, retinopathy, paroxysmal or sustained hypertension, congestive heart failure, pulmonary edema, polycythemia, glycosuria, abdominal pain, vomiting, polydipsia, polyuria, diabetes mellitus, loss of subcutaneous fat and an elevated basal metabolic rate. These symptoms are the result of catecholamines elaborated by the tumor. Techniques have been developed for assay of the pressor amines epinephrine and norepinephrine and of the metabolites such as VMA and HMMA in the urine and body fluids. Occasionally, these tumors may secrete or be associated with increased hydrocortisone or high thyroidal uptake of I^{131}.

In patients with paroxysmal elevation of blood pressure, hypertension can often be induced by massage of the costovertebral angle or injection of histamine, tyramine, tetraethylammonium chloride or mecholyl. If hypertension is adrenergic, blocking agents such as phenyltoloxamine will often lower the pressure.

Pheochromocytomas may occur in patients with neurofibromatosis, cerebellar hemangioblastoma (Hippel-Lindau disease), hypernephroma, thyroid medullary cancer, parathyroid adenoma and other neoplasms. Pheochromocytoma may be familial (Figs. 85 and 86) and is then often multicentric. More often in young children than in adults, the tumor is multiple.

ROENTGEN CHANGES.—On plain roentgenograms and intravenous urograms, because most pheochromocytomas are relatively large at the time of examination, they may often be seen as a soft tissue mass or diagnosed as a result of displacement of the kidney (Figs. 82, *B*; 85, *A*). In our patients, the tumor averaged 120 Gm, and it was detected without the use of special procedures in about 30%. Calcification of the tumor is not common. It may appear as an amorphous calcific mass or as a shell around an area of cystic degeneration (Fig. 82, *C*).

Extraperitoneal pneumography has been successful at our institution, and 11 of 12 tumors collected a few years ago were diagnosed correctly (Figs. 81–86). Errors in diagnosis may result if the tumor is small, multiple or associated with extra-adrenal neoplasms in the region of the kidney hilus, in the organ of Zuckerkandl (Figs. 87 and 88) or in the pelvis. The tumors are usually oval or spherical. The apex of the remaining uninvolved adrenal gland may appear as a triangular shadow on top of the mass (Fig. 81, *A*). The opposite adrenal is of normal size (Fig. 81, *B* and *C*) unless it contains a tumor, unlike the contralateral atrophic adrenals in Cushing's syndrome.

The probability of successful diagnosis of extra-adrenal neoplasms is greater with arteriography than with extraperitoneal pneumography (Figs. 87 and 88). Arteriograms also are more likely to show additional neoplasms lying outside the adrenal. Aortography or selective adrenal arteriography may be applied in the same manner as in Cushing's syndrome. The tumors are often highly vascular. Deaths have been reported from aortography, but if the blood pressure and the heart rate are monitored during the procedure, appropriate adrenergic agents may be administered immediately a change is noted.

To summarize, adrenal neoplasms of all types may be seen on plain roentgenograms if the tumors are sufficiently large. Those tumors often attaining large size before producing symptoms, such as virilizing or non-hormone-secreting cortical adenomas and pheochromocytomas, are more often identified. Urograms may aid in demonstrating these tumors and show deviation of the ureter and extrinsic pressure on the bladder produced by extra-adrenal masses. The urogram also reveals displacement of the kidney downward by adrenal neoplasms, or upward or laterally by extra-adrenal lesions. Aldosterone-secreting tumors are usually small and not demonstrated without the use of special techniques.

Extraperitoneal pneumography has its most important application in identifying adrenal cortical adenomas and hyperplasia associated with Cushing's syndrome. These lesions are relatively avascular. Pheochromocytomas are often extremely vascular and are usually readily diagnosed by aortography or selective arteriography.

Adrenal venography has been successful in identifying small aldosterone-secreting tumors not seen by other methods of examination.

Calcification may occur with cortical, medullary or ectopic benign or malignant neoplasms. It is most common in adrenal neuroblastomas.

Figure 58.—Adrenal cyst.

A, intravenous urogram, demonstrating a soft tissue mass somewhat triangular is shape above the superior pole of the kidney. Thin linear calcifications outline the lateral and inferior margins of the mass (**arrows**). The upper pole of the kidney is rotated laterally.

B, extraperitoneal pneumogram, obtained after the injection of gas in the retrorectal extraperitoneal tissues. The mass is outlined by gas (**arrows**). There is no roentgen evidence of a normal adrenal remnant. Note that the contralateral adrenal (**a**) is within normal limits.

The lesion was an adrenal cyst with calcium in its wall. Several similar cases of calcified adrenal cyst have been reported.

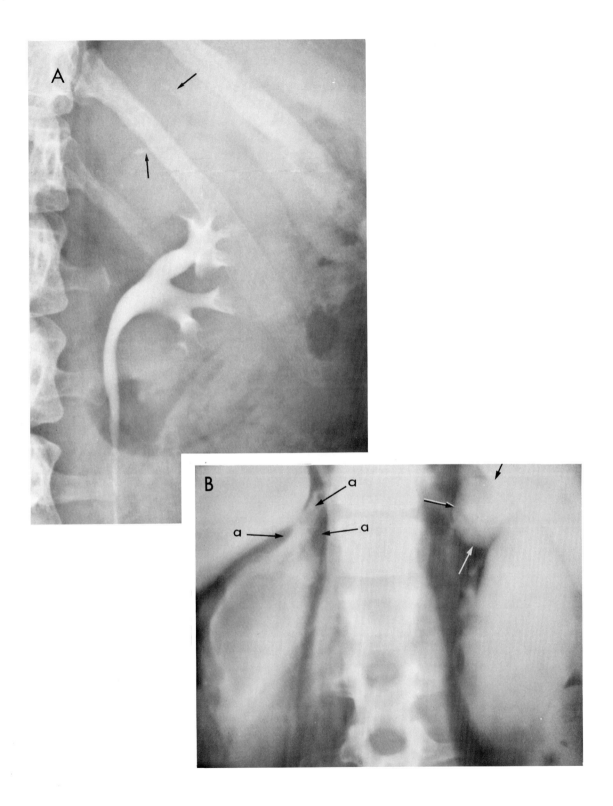

Figure 58 · Adrenal Cyst / 173

Figure 59.—Nonhormonal benign adrenal adenoma (all figures from same patient).

A, left posterior oblique roentgenogram, after oxygen had been injected between the rectum and sacrum. A large tumor, partly outlined by oxygen (**a**), displaces the right kidney caudally and compresses the upper pole (**b**).

B, lateral view, demonstrating the tumor (**a**) and displaced kidney (**b**).

C, aortogram, performed while oxygen was still present in the retroperitoneal area. The tumor is extremely vascular and receives a large vessel probably arising from the inferior phrenic artery (**c**) and a large adrenal artery arising from the aorta near the origin of the renal artery (**d**). The renal artery is stretched (**e**).

The patient was being investigated because of hypertension. Urinary levels of catecholamines, 17-ketosteroids and 17-hydroxycorticoids were normal. The pathologic diagnosis was adrenal cortical adenoma. The blood pressure became normal following its removal. The hypertension probably resulted from compression of the upper pole of the kidney or branches of the renal artery.

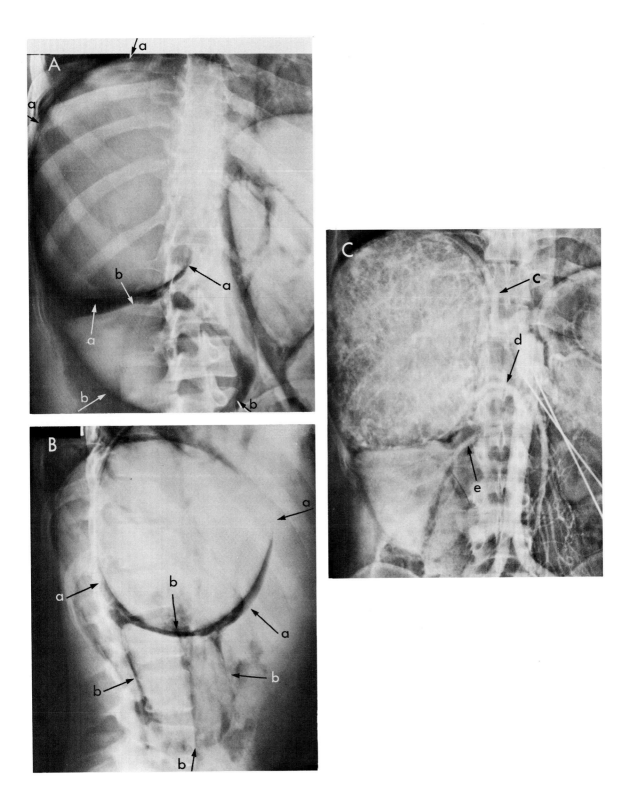

Figure 59 · Cortical Adenoma / 175

Figure 60.—Adrenal cortical adenoma.

A, anteroposterior roentgenogram of the hands and wrists of a 2½-year-old girl, showing the pisiform bone in each wrist. The pisiforms normally appear at about age 10.

B, left posterior oblique 10-minute intravenous urogram, revealing depression of the superior margin of the right kidney and a zone of demarcation between a soft tissue mass and the kidney (**arrow**).

The patient was seen for study because of sudden development of a voracious appetite, rapid weight gain and signs of sexual maturation. At operation, the adrenal gland containing a large cortical adenoma was removed.

Figure 60, courtesy of Hope, J. W., and Koop, C. E.: M. Photog. & Radiog., vol. 38, no. 1, 1962.

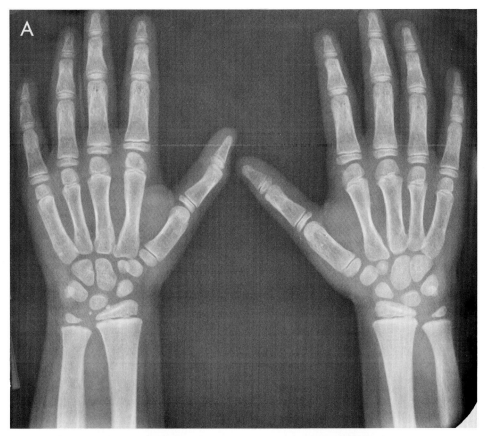

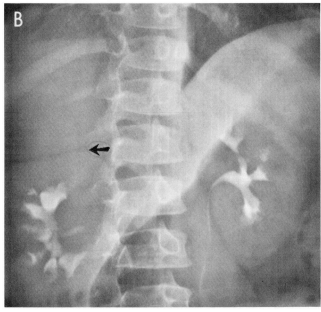

Figure 60 · Cortical Adenoma / 177

Figure 61.—Aldosterone-secreting adrenal cortical tumor.

This patient had a history of hypertension. On one test, the blood aldosterone level was normal, but another indicated an elevated blood aldosterone value, prompting adrenal roentgen studies.

Adrenal phlebogram: Revealing a tumor stain in the left adrenal (**x**). At operation, two small adenomas were found within the adrenal gland and were removed.

Figure 61, courtesy of Dr. S. R. Reuter, Eloise, Mich.

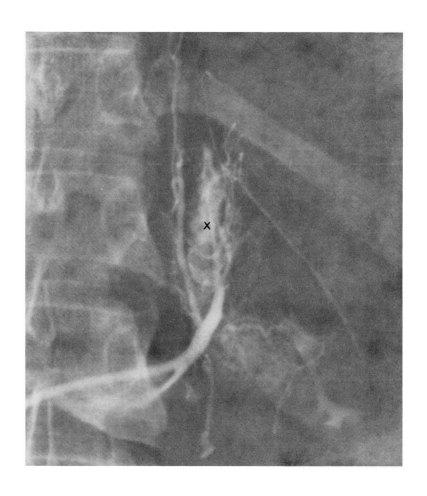

Figure 61 · Aldosterone-secreting Adrenal Tumor / 179

Figure 62.—Aldosterone-secreting adrenal cortical tumor.

A, body section study after retroperitoneal air injection: Revealing a normal left adrenal (**arrow**). The right adrenal (**arrow**) was also normal. The tumor, in actual fact, was situated on the upper pole of the left kidney at **x**.

B (same patient as in *A*), phlebogram of left adrenal vein: Revealing the blush of a group of tumor vessels (**arrows**) identifying the adrenal adenoma. It was removed surgically and measured slightly less than 2 cm in diameter.

Figure 62, courtesy of Dr. Koson Kuroda, Philadelphia.

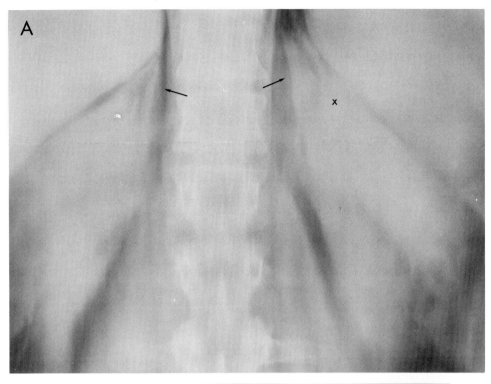

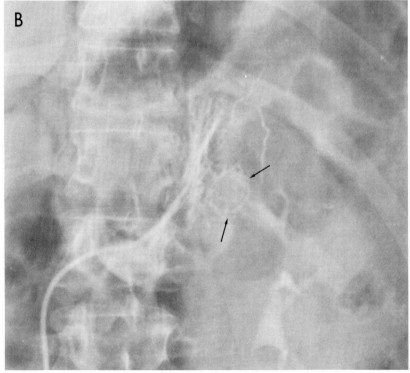

Figure 62 · Aldosterone-secreting Adrenal Tumor / 181

Figure 63.—Cushing's syndrome resulting from benign adrenal adenoma.

A, tomogram after oxygen was introduced into the retroperitoneal tissues between the rectum and sacrum under controlled pressure. The gas has passed cranially to outline the psoas shadows (**a**), kidneys (**b**) and adrenals.

A small mass is visible above the left kidney in the space usually occupied by the adrenal gland (**c**). The mass is oval, with the apex pointed. The left kidney has not been displaced or distorted. The opposite adrenal is atrophic (**d**). It has the shape of an elongated triangle and its margins are slightly concave.

The tumor was an adenoma, in a patient with Cushing's syndrome.

B, tomogram, showing a moderate-sized adenoma of the left adrenal outlined by gas (**a**). The left kidney has been displaced downward and is slightly rotated (**b**). The left kidney is higher than the right in about 90% of normal individuals. The apex of the adrenal tumor is triangular, representing normal adrenal tissue. The lower part of the adrenal has been replaced by the spherical mass which blends with the remaining normal triangular adrenal tissue above.

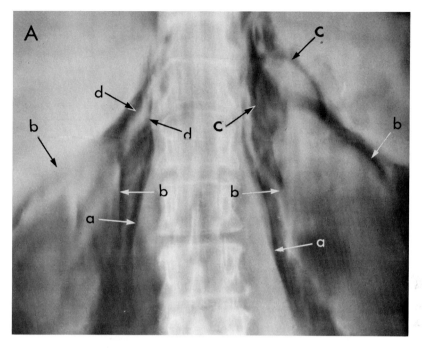

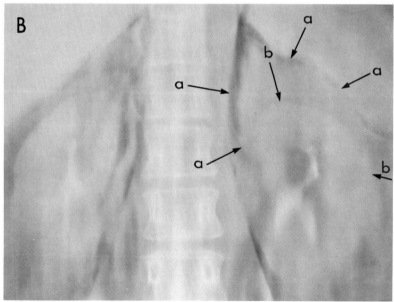

Figure 63 · Cushing's Syndrome from Adenoma / 183

Figure 64.—Cushing's syndrome resulting from benign adrenal adenoma.

A, tomogram after gas injection. The adrenals are not well outlined by the gas, which has not yet penetrated the overlying fat. The left adrenal (**a**) appears to be larger than the right (**b**).

B, roentgenogram obtained later, showing the small left adrenal adenoma sharply outlined by gas (**a**). The lumbar vertebrae are osteoporotic, with diminished density and thin compact bone. A fracture has occurred in the twelfth vertebral body, depressing the superior plate (**c**).

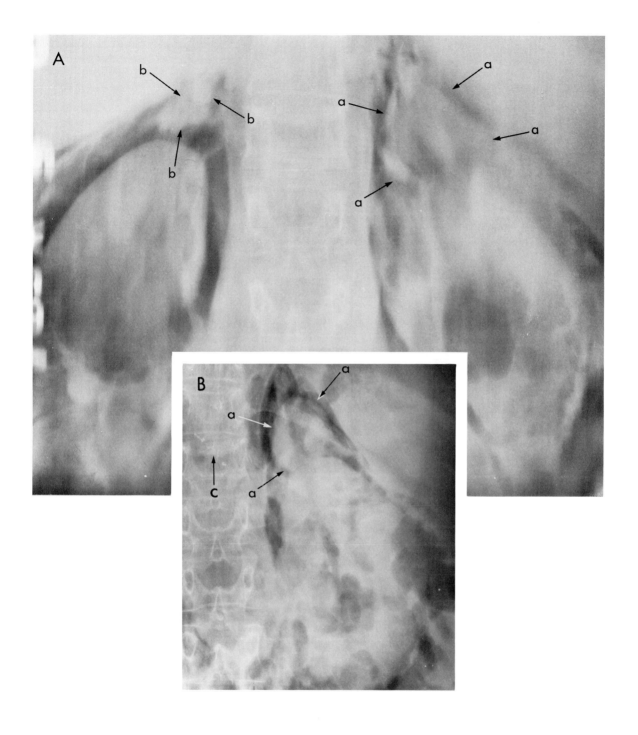

Figure 64 · Cushing's Syndrome from Adenoma / 185

Figure 65.—Cushing's syndrome resulting from benign adrenal adenoma.

A, tomogram, demonstrating a large cortical adenoma (**a**). The mass is located above the right kidney and is almost spherical.

B, tomogram after extraperitoneal pneumography, showing the large mass well outlined (**a**). The upper pole of the kidney appears to be slightly flattened. The left adrenal is not outlined by the gas.

C, early stage of an aortogram, anteroposterior projection. The vascularity of the tumor is minimally increased. A relatively large adrenal artery (**b**) extends from the aorta toward the adrenal mass, giving off several smaller branches.

D, right posterior oblique projection. The roentgenogram, exposed at a later interval following the injection of contrast material, shows smaller branches of the adrenal artery feeding the upper part of the adenoma (**c**).

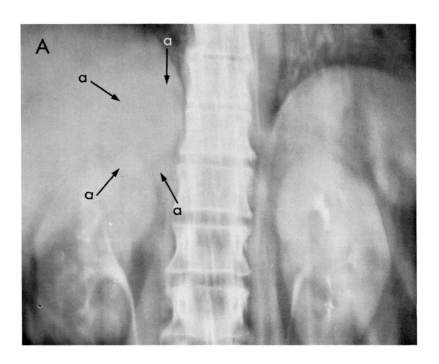

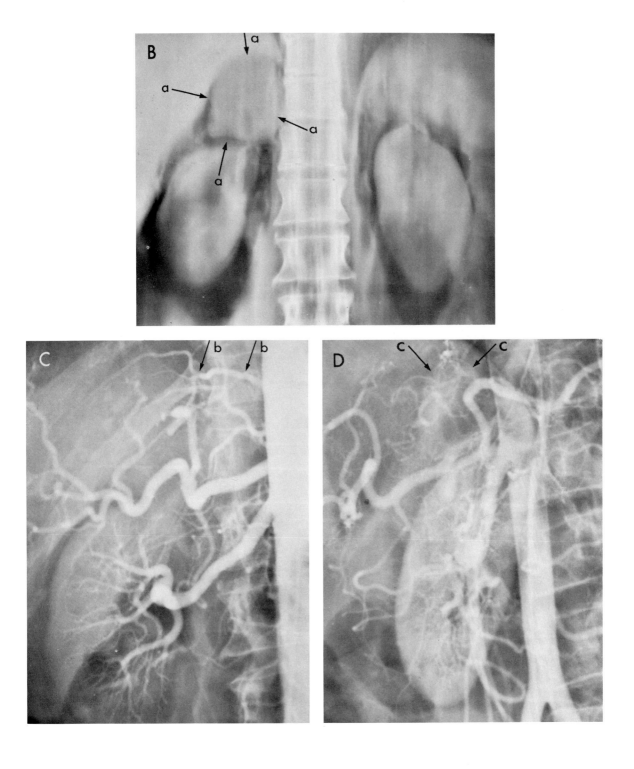

Figure 65 · Cushing's Syndrome from Adenoma / 187

Figure 66.—Cushing's syndrome resulting from benign adrenal adenoma.

A, extraperitoneal pneumogram, showing a large cortical adenoma of the right adrenal (a). The gland retains some of its triangular shape, although the lateral margins are convex rather than straight or concave, as is usually seen in the normal adrenal. The left adrenal is atrophic and cannot be separated from the surrounding fatty connective tissue (b). The right kidney is displaced downward by the adenoma and is rotated along its vertical axis (c).

B, intravenous urogram, demonstrating a very large right adrenal cortical adenoma (a). The right kidney is displaced downward and rotated on its longitudinal axis by the adenoma. The tumor has rounded borders and is approaching the contour of a sphere. Several small rounded or oval calcific densities are seen within it (b).

C, tomogram of the right side, better demonstrating the mass (a) and calcification (b) within it.

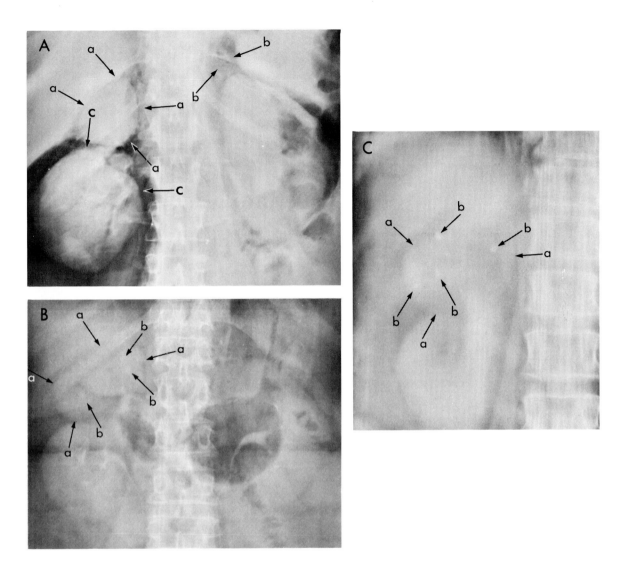

Figure 66 · Cushing's Syndrome from Adenoma / 189

Figure 67.—Cushing's syndrome resulting from benign adrenal adenoma.

A, intravenous urogram, showing the left kidney displaced cranially and compressed by a huge mass (**a**) which overlies the lower half of the kidney and extends caudally almost to the innominate bone. The calices of the lower pole of the kidney are distorted, and the ureter (**b**) is compressed and displaced toward the spine. As with many other retroperitoneal tumors, the shadow normally cast by the psoas muscle has been partially obliterated. The adenoma has arisen in aberrant adrenal tissue.

B, tomogram, showing a very large right adrenal mass (**a**) displacing the kidney caudally. The mass is oval and contains a small calcific density laterally (**b**).

C, aortogram (same patient as in *B*), showing the mass to be extremely vascular. Large adrenal vessels arise from the right renal artery and supply the inferior portion of the tumor (**c**). Other smaller vessels coming directly from the aorta supply the superior and medial portions of the tumor (**d**).

The tumor was interpreted by the pathologist as a very cellular cortical adenoma of questionable malignancy.

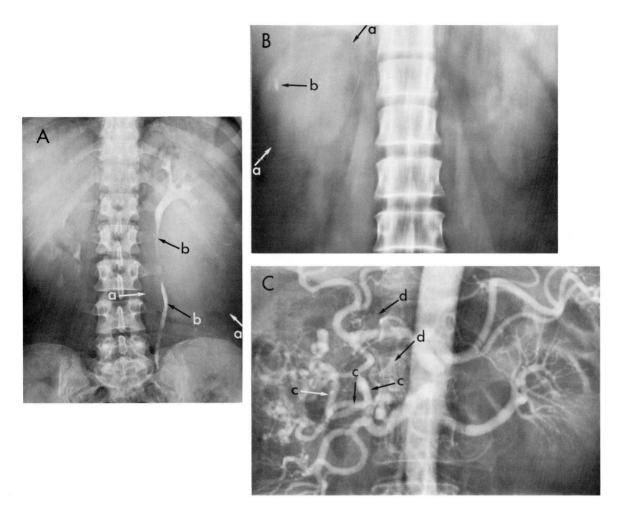

Figure 67 · Cushing's Syndrome from Adenoma / 191

Figure 68.—Cushing's syndrome resulting from adrenal carcinoma.

Extraperitoneal pneumogram of a 13½-year-old boy with typical Cushing's syndrome. The tomogram reveals a moderately enlarged, well-delineated right adrenal gland (**a**). The adrenal retains its triangular appearance, but the margins are convex. A normal adrenal has straight or concave margins. The left adrenal is atrophic (**b**).

The vertebrae are demineralized. The superior borders of the tenth and eleventh vertebral bodies are depressed and there is an increased density beneath the end-plates (**c**), as is often seen in Cushing's syndrome. The skeletal age, estimated from roentgenograms of the hand, was 10 years, indicating that the disease had been present for more than 4 years.

The resected adrenal gland was 3.5 cm in diameter and weighed 9 Gm. Cellular pleomorphism and loss of normal architecture were noted microscopically. The tumor did not invade the capsule or blood vessels. Diagnosis was adrenocortical carcinoma.

The patient, followed for several years, had no recurrence. Adrenal tumors of Cushing's syndrome in children are often malignant.

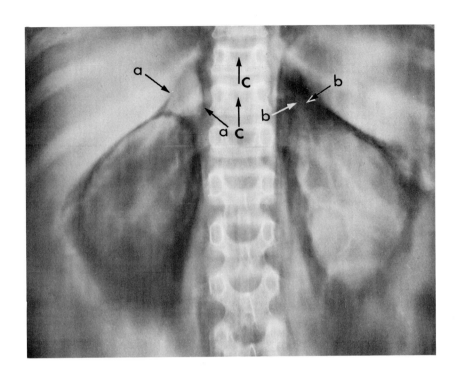

Figure 68 · Cushing's Syndrome from Carcinoma / 193

Figure 69.—Cushing's syndrome resulting from adrenal carcinoma (all figures from same patient).

A, intravenous urogram, showing a huge mass arising in the left adrenal (**a**) and displacing the kidney caudally. The intrarenal structures appear to be normal.

B, extraperitoneal pneumogram, outlining the inferior and lateral margins of the spherical tumor (**a**). The lower pole of the kidney is visible below the tumor (**b**). The transverse colon (**c**) and stomach (**d**) contain gas and are displaced cranially.

C, roentgenogram of a gastrointestinal series, showing displacement of the stomach cranially and to the right (**d**). The retroperitoneal portion of the duodenum is displaced to the right, and the jejunum to the right and caudally (**e**).

D, lateral view of the gastrointestinal series, demonstrating the mass behind the stomach (**d**) and small bowel and displacing it ventrally (**f**).

Diagnosis was adrenal cortical carcinoma.

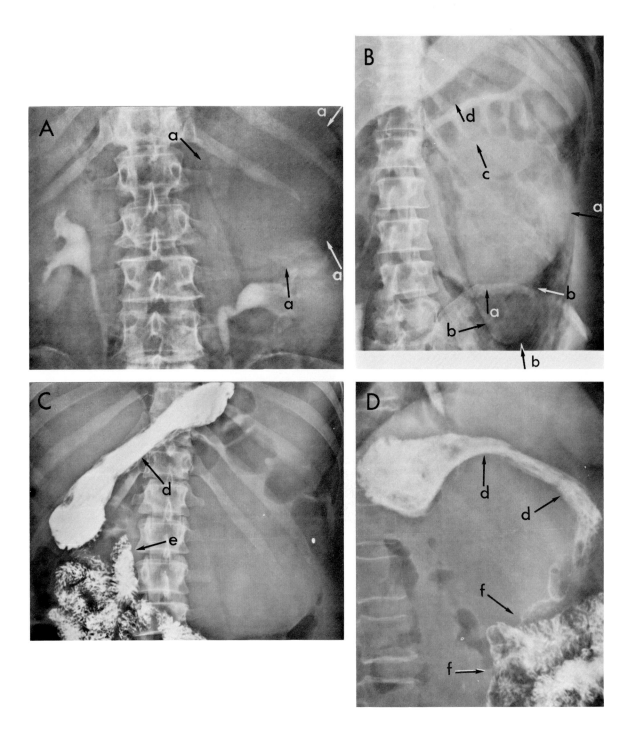

Figure 69 · Cushing's Syndrome from Carcinoma / 195

Figure 70.—Virilizing unilateral adrenal tumors.

A, extraperitoneal pneumogram. The gas has not penetrated the space between the right kidney and adrenal (**a**). The left adrenal is visible, however, and not enlarged (**b**). Diagnosis was right adrenal cortical adenoma.

B, intravenous urogram. A large mass displaces the left kidney caudally and rotates it along its longitudinal axis. Within the mass are fine interlacing strands and coarse amorphous calcifications (**arrows**). This was an adrenal adenocarcinoma.

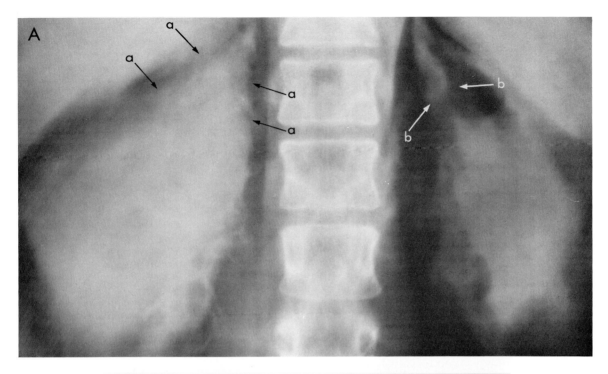

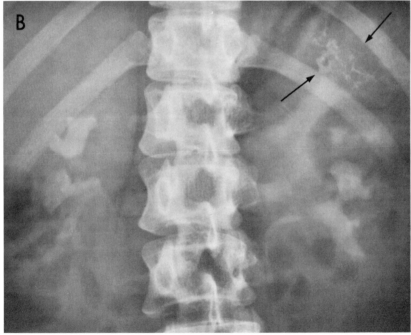

Figure 70 · Virilizing Unilateral Tumor / 197

Figure 71.—Virilizing unilateral adrenal adneocarcinoma.

Extraperitoneal pneumogram, revealing a very large tumor (**a**) displacing the kidney caudally and rotating it (**b**). The remnant of the adrenal gland is visible as a triangular shadow above the mass (**c**).

The patient had had progressive hirsutism for 2 years. At operation, the tumor, measuring 9 cm in diameter and weighing 110 Gm, was removed. There was focal capsular invasion by neoplastic cells and extension into the walls of vascular channels. The diagnosis was adrenal cortical adenocarcinoma.

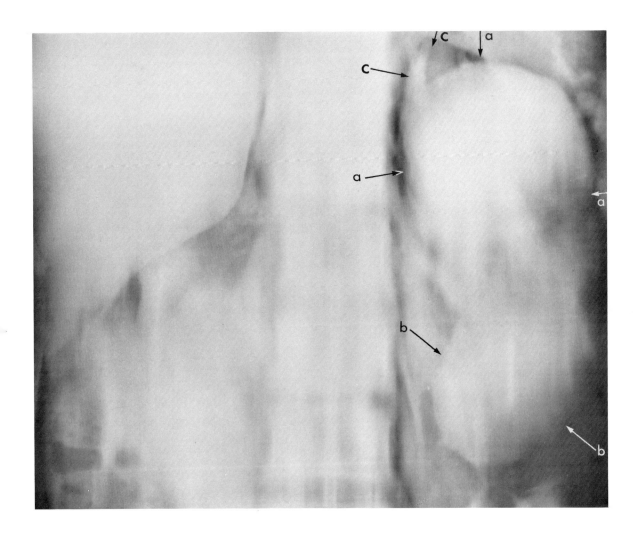

Figure 71 · Virilizing Unilateral Tumor / 199

Figure 72.—Osteoporosis resulting from Cushing's syndrome.

A, lateral roentgenogram of the lumbar region, revealing demineralization of the vertebral bodies. Compression fractures of the upper and lower end-plates have occurred. There are homogeneous dense horizontal bands just beneath the end-plates (**arrows**), which are seen often in cases of Cushing's syndrome and rarely with other forms of osteoporosis.

B, lateral roentgenogram, obtained 1 year after treatment, reveals continuing osteoporosis which will probably persist. Almost all of the horizontal dense bands have disappeared. The osteoporosis may not now be differentiated from that caused by postmenopausal or senile osteoporosis.

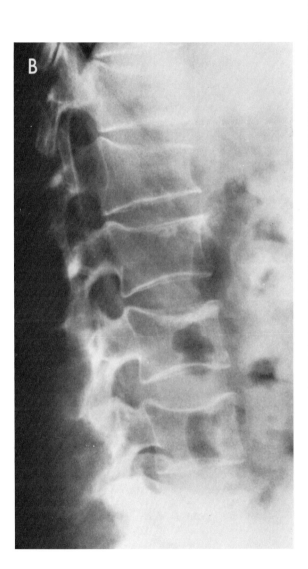

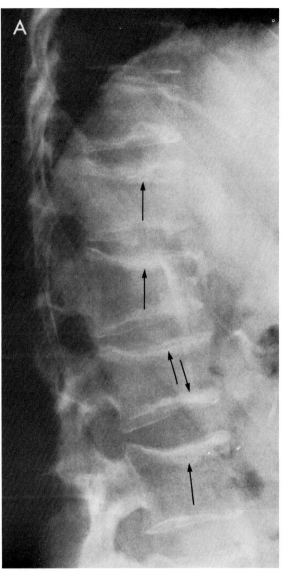

Figure 72 · Cushing's Syndrome: Osteoporosis / 201

Figure 73.—Neuroblastoma.

A, survey roentgenogram, showing upward displacement of the right hemidiaphragm (**arrows**) by a huge mass in the right upper quadrant. Note the fine amorphous deposit of calcium within the mass (**x**).

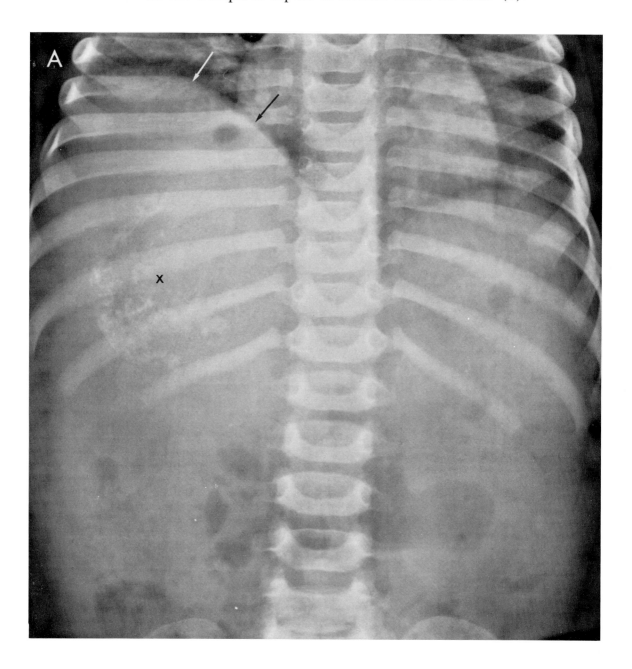

B, anteroposterior intravenous urogram, demonstrating downward displacement of the right kidney with the upper pole tilted laterally. The architecture of the pelvocalyceal collecting system is not distorted, indicating that the mass is extrinsic to the kidney.

The tumor was proved to be a neuroblastoma.

Figure 73, courtesy of Hope, J. W., and Koop, C. E.: M. Radiog. & Photog., vol. 38, no. 1, 1962.

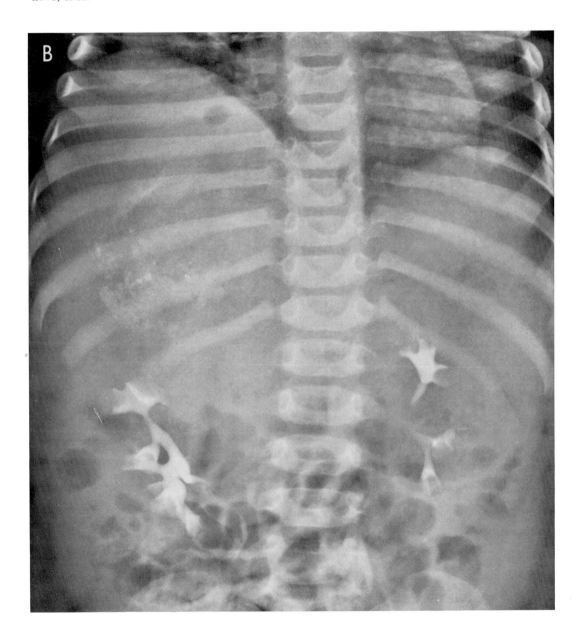

Figure 73 · Neuroblastoma / 203

Figure 74.—Neuroblastoma at the level of the lower pole of the kidney.

A, survey roentgenogram, showing a vertical streak of calcification and small round calcification (**arrows**) to the left of the spine at the level of the second and third lumbar vertebrae. There is an impression of a large, vague soft tissue mass (**x**) in this area that could be palpated in the abdomen.

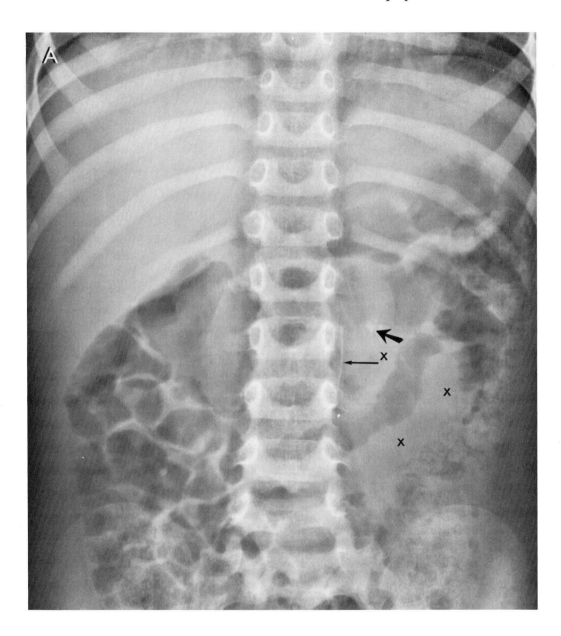

B, anteroposterior intravenous urogram, demonstrating rotation of the left kidney and lateral displacement of its lower pole. Calcification (**arrow**) is present in the soft tissue mass, which is delineated by the proximal ureter. At operation, a neuroblastoma was found that contained calcific debris.

Figure 74, courtesy of Hope, J. W., and Koop, C. E.: M. Radiog. & Photog., vol. 38, no. 1, 1962.

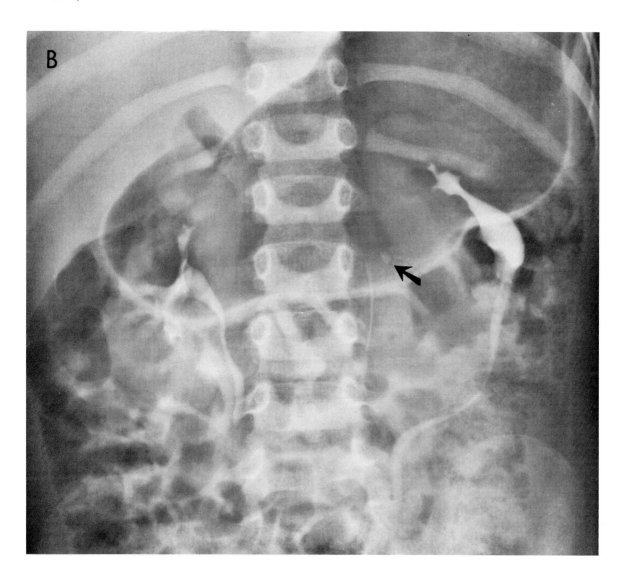

Figure 74 · Neuroblastoma / 205

Figure 75.—Neuroblastoma below the kidney.

A, survey roentgenogram, demonstrating a vague bulge (**arrow**) in the left lower iliopsoas region.

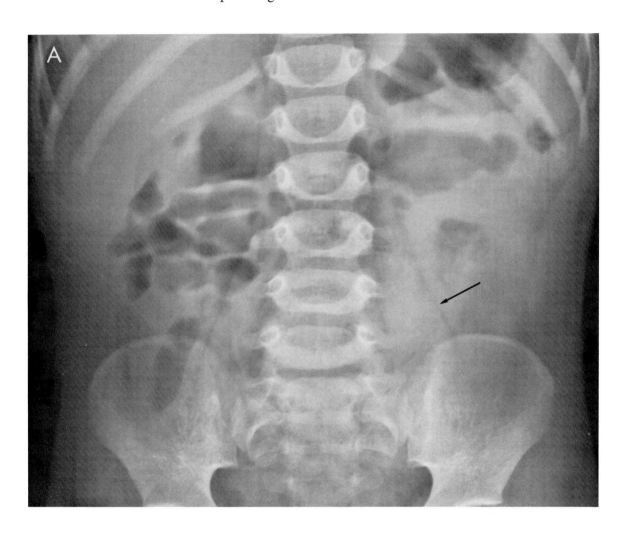

B, anteroposterior 15-minute intravenous urogram, showing medial displacement of the left ureter (**arrow**), which outlines the retroperitoneal mass. The tumor was proved to be a neuroblastoma.

Figure 75, courtesy of Hope, J. W., and Koop, C. E.: M. Radiog. & Photog., vol. 38, no. 1, 1962.

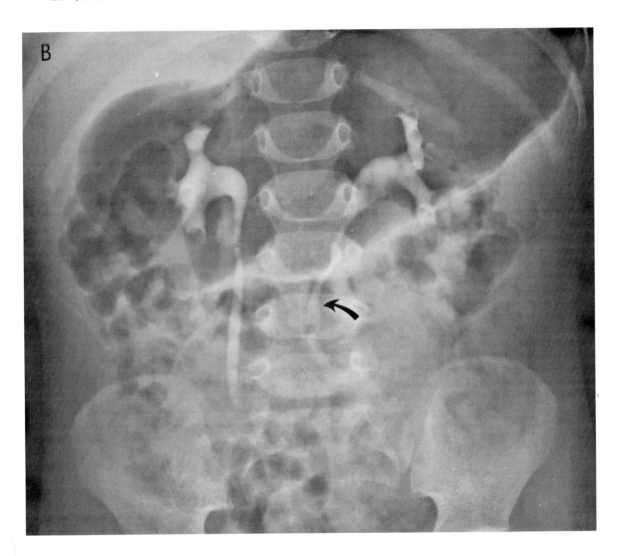

Figure 75 · Neuroblastoma / **207**

Figure 76.—Neuroblastoma producing extrinsic pressure on the bladder.

A, anteroposterior 10-minute intravenous urogram, showing an indentation on the left side of the dome of the bladder (**arrows**).

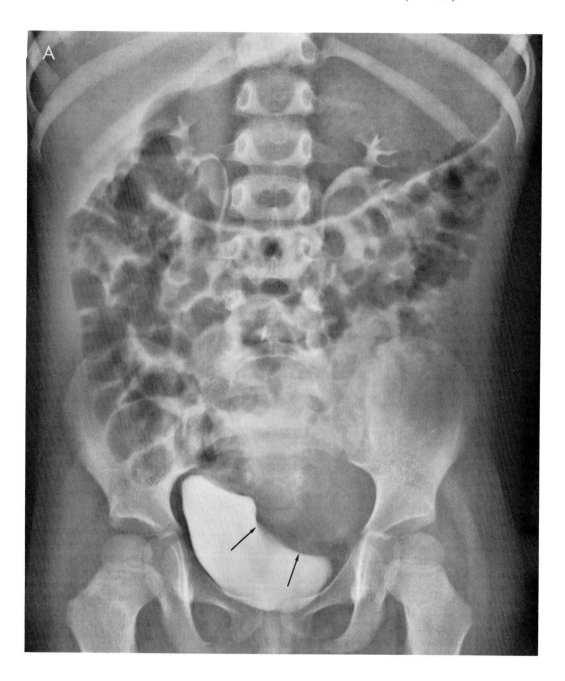

B, anteroposterior 20-minute intravenous urogram, showing medial displacement of the left ureter (**arrows**) by a mass in the left lower quadrant.

The tumor was a pelvic neuroblastoma.

Figure 76, courtesy of Hope, J. W., and Koop, C. E.: M. Radiog. & Photog., vol. 38, no. 1, 1962.

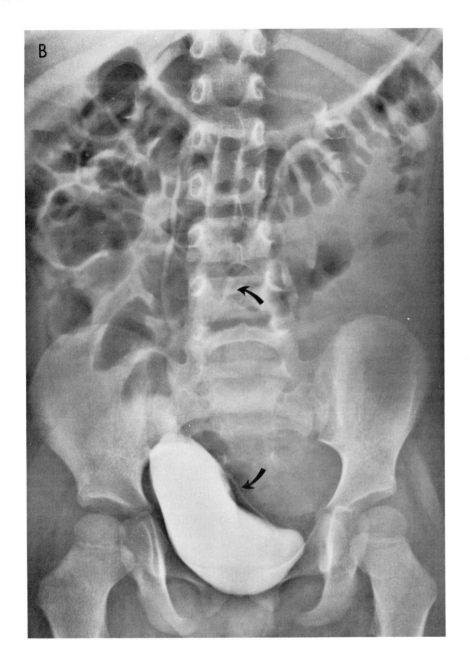

Figure 76 · Neuroblastoma / 209

Figure 77.—Neuroblastoma arising from the organ of Zuckerkandl.

A, survey roentgenogram, showing what appears to be a large left lobe of the liver (**x**) indenting the lesser curvature of the stomach (**arrows**). The entire stomach seems to be displaced to the left. The right lobe of the liver extends to the pelvic bone.

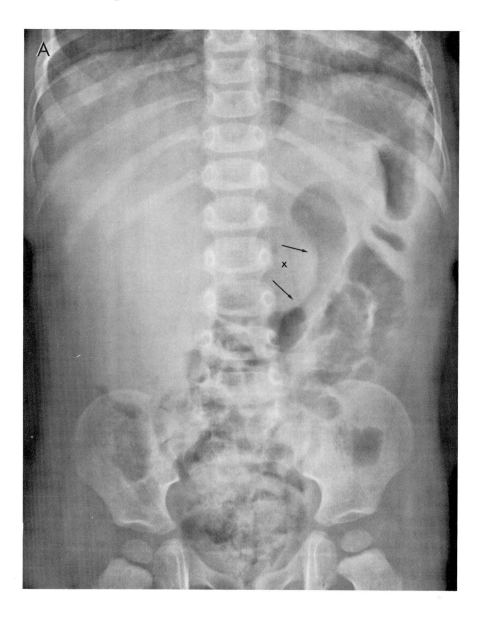

B, anteroposterior 30-minute intravenous roentgenogram, demonstrating no displacement of the left kidney by a tumor. The right pelvocalyceal collecting system contains less opaque material than the left. Because the latter often occurs when the liver is enlarged and pushed backward on the kidney (displacing the kidney posteriorly), the tumor was thought to lie in the liver rather than in the retroperitoneal space (which would displace the kidney anteriorly).

At operation, the mass was found to be a huge neuroblastoma arising from the organ of Zuckerkandl.

Figure 77, courtesy of Hope, J. W., and Koop, C. E.: M. Radiog. & Photog., vol. 38, no. 1, 1962.

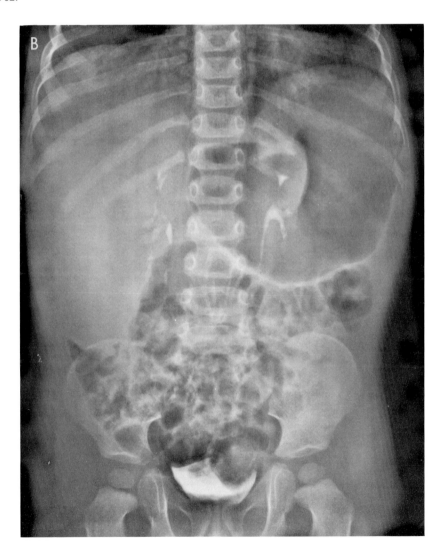

Figure 77 · Neuroblastoma in Organ of Zuckerkandl / 211

Figure 78.—Neuroblastoma with metastases.

A, intravenous urogram of a 3-year-old girl. Small stippled calcific densities are present in the left upper abdomen (**a**). The calcifications are above and lateral to the kidney, with some superimposed on its upper pole. A distinct soft tissue mass is not visible. Numerous osteolytic (destructive) lesions are visible in the pelvis and upper portions of the femurs. Scattered about are osteoblastic areas, best seen adjacent to the apophysis for the greater trochanter (**b**).

B, anteroposterior view, showing the lytic lesions to be very small and streaky because of the infiltrative nature of the malignancy. Most of the trabeculae are spared, and some are thickened and sclerotic, particularly in the upper and lower parts of the femur and the upper left tibia (**b**). A thin shell of periosteal new bone is visible around the distal third of the right femur (**c**). The epiphyses are not obviously involved. Characteristic features are the bilateral symmetry and infiltration. Lymphosarcoma and leukemia may cause a similar appearance.

C, roentgenogram of the resected tumor. The calcifications are clearly visible. The tumor is larger than the calcifications on the urogram (**a**) suggested.

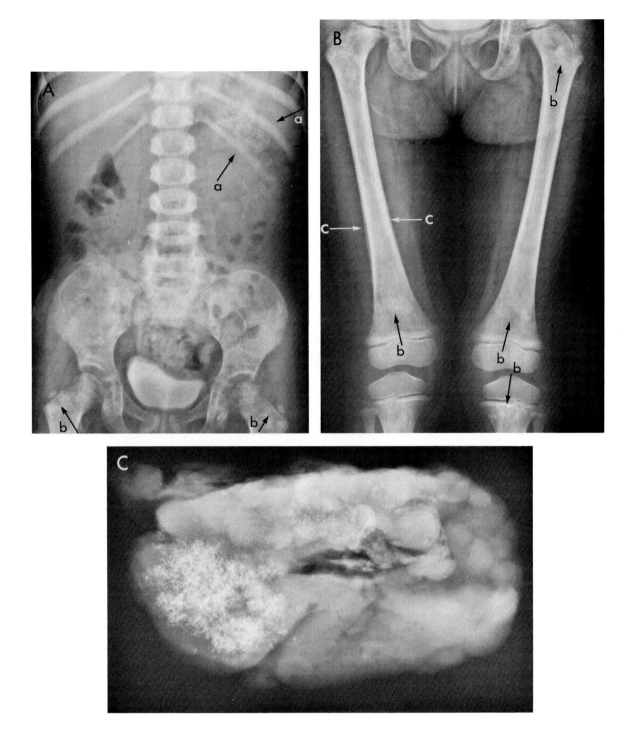

Figure 78 · Neuroblastoma: Metastases / 213

Figure 79.—Neuroblastoma with metastases.

A, survey abdominal exposure of a 4-year-old girl. Small linear and punctate calcific densities are scattered throughout a mass which extends from the level of the ninth thoracic to the fifth lumbar vertebra and from the left abdominal wall to the right of the spine (**a**). The liver is large (**b**) and has displaced the large right kidney caudally. The tumor has extended along the spine into the mediastinum (**c**).

B, anteroposterior roentgenogram, showing an unusual response to the metastatic neoplasm. The distal ends of the femurs are widened and the cortex is thinned. The appearance is similar to that which occurs from bone marrow involvement by relatively benign diseases, such as Gaucher's and hyperplasia of marrow secondary to hemolytic anemia. Sharply delineated spicules of bone radiate from the center of the shaft. These probably represent the path of spread of the tumor, which has stimulated periosteal bone formation. Above this, on the left side is an oval radiolucent lesion.

A biopsy of the bone lesion revealed that the neuroblastoma had matured to form ganglioneuroma.

C, posteroanterior, and **D,** lateral roentgenograms, revealing the same type of radiating bone spicules as seen in the femur, here involving the facial bones (**d**) and frontal bone (**e**). A similar process is present in the right parietal bone (**f**). The facial bones are small and the interorbital distance is diminished (hypotelorism), probably as a result of the adverse effect of the neoplasm on the growth process. The coronal sutures are wide, with long serrations (**g**), and the floor of the anterior fossa is depressed because of increased intracranial pressure.

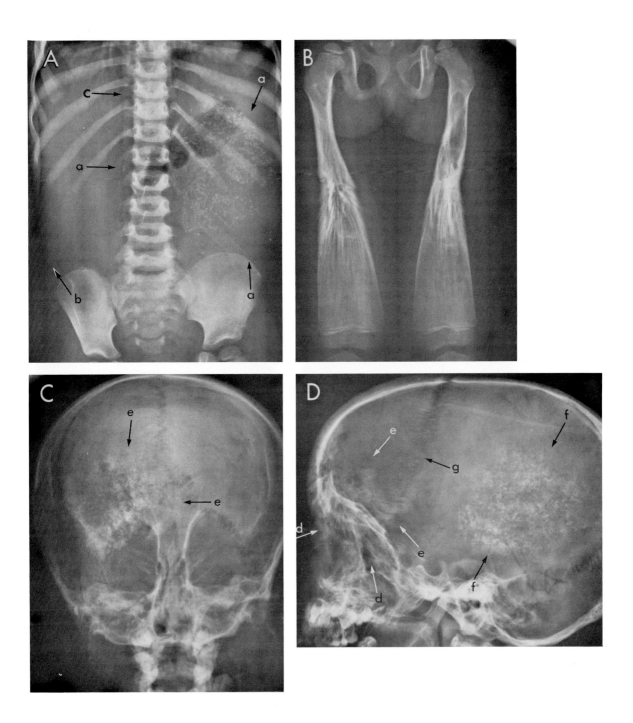

Figure 79 · Neuroblastoma: Metastases / 215

Figure 80.—Metastases from neuroblastoma.

A, lateral view of the skull of a 4-year-old boy. A mottled rarefaction involves the frontal bones, outer third of the parietal and occipital bones, the anterior part of the base of the skull and the facial bones. The cranium is large in size due to widening of the coronal and sagittal sutures and, to a lesser extent, the lambdoidal suture. This indicates increased intracranial pressure, most likely from infiltration of neoplastic cells beneath the dura mater. The bony margins of the coronal suture have large serrations. Spicules of bone extend at right angles to the calvarium into the soft tissues, as demonstrated on the inset (**arrows**).

B, anteroposterior view, showing mixed radiolucent (**a**) and sclerotic lesions (**b**) extending through the pelvis and shafts of both femurs. The radiolucent lesions predominate and are small, with punctate areas in the spongy bone, whereas others are linear in the cortex. The disease is almost bilaterally symmetrical.

The diagnosis was sympathicoblastoma of the left adrenal gland.

Figure 80, courtesy of Grier, G. W.: Radiog. & Clin. Photog. 20:50, 1944.

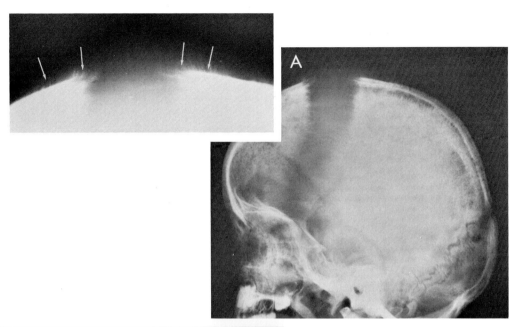

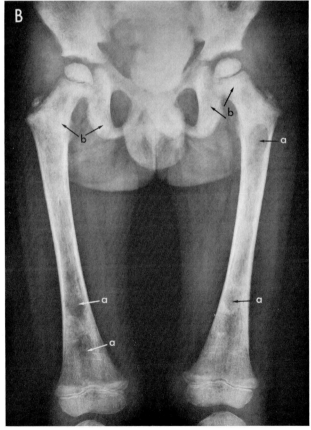

Figure 80 · Neuroblastoma: Metastases / 217

Figure 81.—Pheochromocytoma.

A, tomogram of an extraperitoneal pneumogram, demonstrating a relatively small pheochromocytoma of the right adrenal (**arrows**). Cranial to the mass is a triangular shadow (**a**) that probably represents normal cortical tissues. Pheochromocytomas are usually large tumors and are not difficult to diagnose by this method if they arise in the adrenal.

B, tomogram of an extraperitoneal pneumogram, showing a moderate-sized pheochromocytoma superimposed on the upper pole of the left kidney (**a**). The right adrenal is normal (**b**).

C, tomogram of an extraperitoneal pneumogram, showing a large lobulated pheochromocytoma lying partly craniad and partly ventral to the left kidney (**a**), which is in its normal position. The right adrenal is normal (**b**).

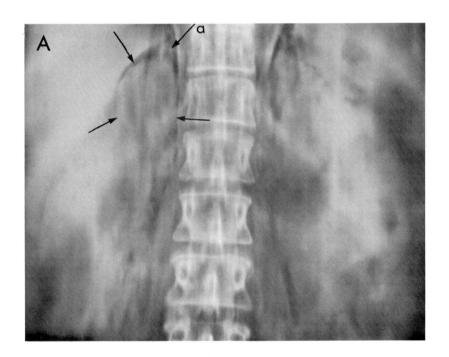

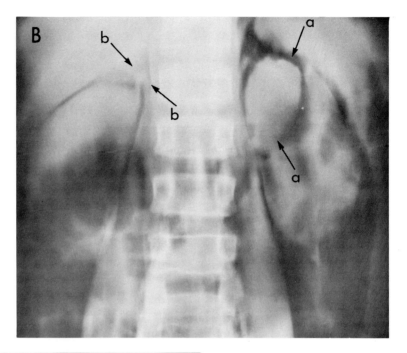

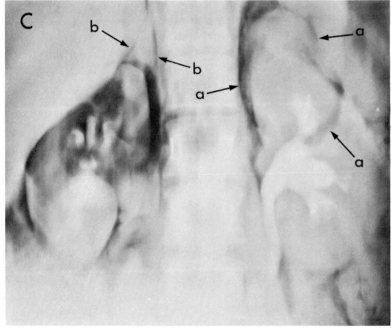

Figure 81 · Pheochromocytoma / 219

Figure 82.—Pheochromocytoma.

A, tomogram of an extraperitoneal pneumogram. A large spherical pheochromocytoma (**arrows**) compresses the upper pole of the left kidney and displaces it caudally. Normal adrenal tissue is visible as a triangular shadow above the tumor.

B, intravenous urogram, revealing a moderate-sized spherical mass superimposed over the upper pole of the kidney and cranial to it (**arrows**).

C, tomogram showing the mass faintly outlined (**a**) and a curved linear calcification (**b**) along its lower margin. This may be in the capsule.

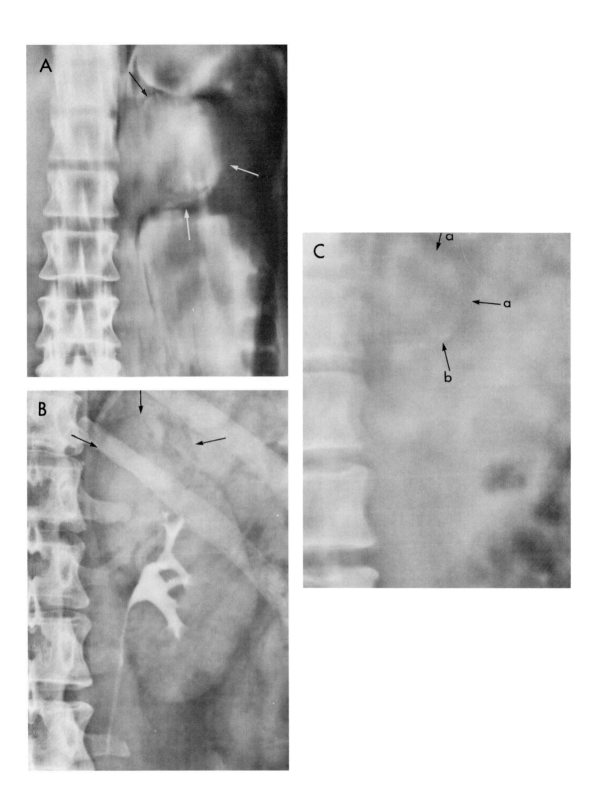

Figure 82 · Pheochromocytoma / 221

Figure 83.—Pheochromocytoma.

Tomogram of an extraperitoneal pneumogram, showing a large mass above the upper pole of the right kidney (**arrows**).

This patient had neurofibromatosis. In patients with neurofibromatosis, pheochromocytomas as well as other neoplasms may develop.

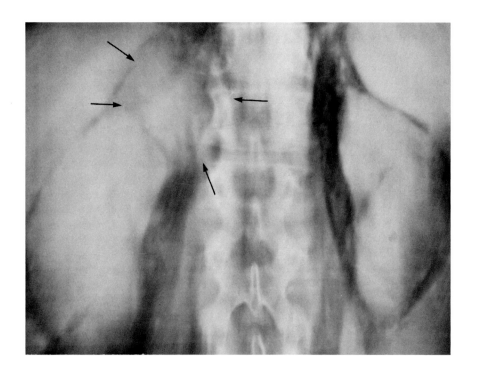

Figure 83 · Pheochromocytoma / 223

Figure 84.—Pheochromocytoma.

A, anteroposterior 5-minute intravenous urogram, disclosing severe dilatation of all of the calices on the left side and no evidence of the renal pelvis (**arrows**). A right posterior oblique 10-minute urogram (not shown) revealed a definite filling defect in the left renal hilus, apparently caused by a mass obliterating the left renal pelvis.

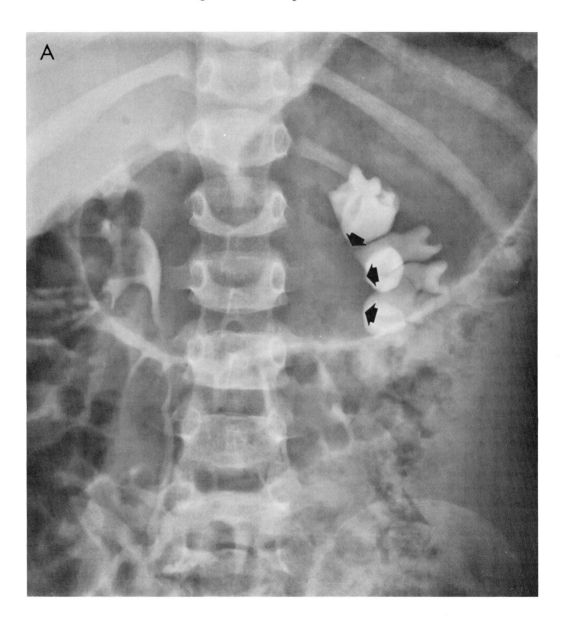

B, anteroposterior roentgenogram following left presacral injection of air (**a**) into the retroperitoneal space, clearly outlining a mass in the left renal hilus (**arrows**).

Figure 84, courtesy of Hope, J. W., and Koop, C. E.: M. Radiog. & Photog., vol. 38, no. 1, 1962.

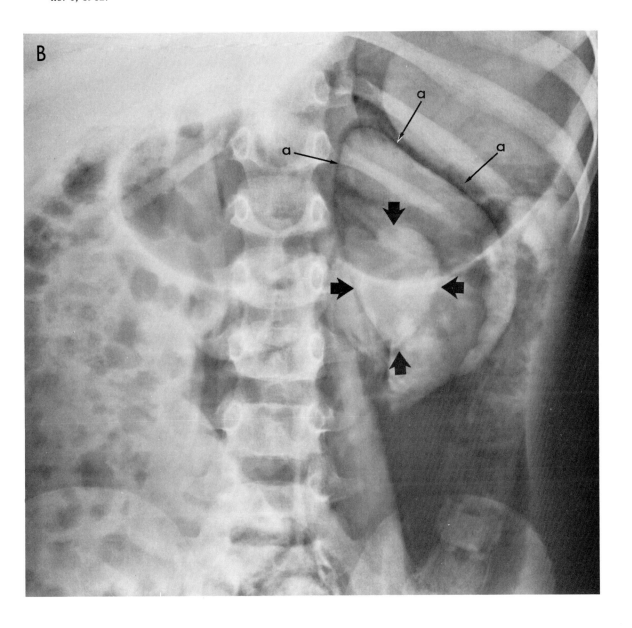

Figure 84 · Pheochromocytoma / 225

Figure 85.—Familial pheochromocytoma.

A, plain roentgenogram of the abdomen of a 20-year-old youth. A small spherical mass is visible in front of and above the upper pole of the right kidney (**arrows**). This tumor could be easily missed if one were not looking for it.

B, tomogram of an extraperitoneal pneumogram. The right adrenal tumor (**arrows**) is better demonstrated here than on the plain roentgenogram (*A*). The triangular portion of the adrenal cortex is above the tumor.

(*Continued* in Figure 86.)

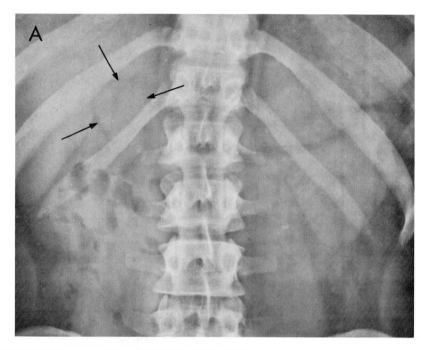

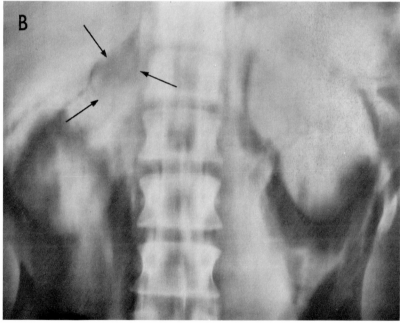

Figure 85 · Familial Pheochromocytoma / 227

Figure 86.—Familial pheochromocytoma.

These radiographs are of the sister of the patient described in Figure 85.

A, extraperitoneal pneumogram, obtained when the patient was 17 years old. There is a huge spherical pheochromocytoma cranial to the left kidney (**a**) and displacing it caudally (**b**). The right adrenal gland is not well demonstrated.

B, intravenous urogram obtained 10 years after the pheochromocytoma of the left adrenal gland had been removed. A large mass in the region of the right adrenal (**a**) displaces the kidney caudally (**b**).

C, extraperitoneal pneumogram, revealing the right pheochromocytoma outlined by gas (**arrows**).

The father of these two patients died of a cerebrovascular accident and at autopsy was found to have bilateral pheochromocytomas. When these tumors occur in families, they are often multiple and may become apparent at an early age.

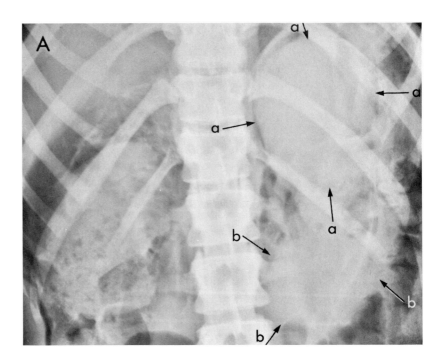

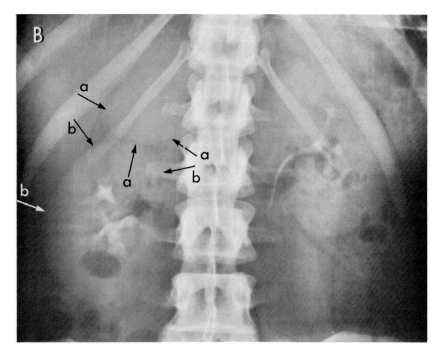

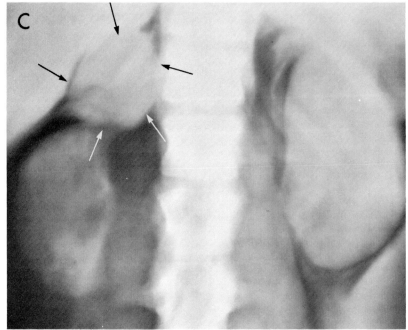

Figure 86 · Familial Pheochromocytoma / 229

Figure 87.—Extra-adrenal pheochromocytoma arising from the organ of Zuckerkandl.

A, intravenous urogram, showing the left ureter deviated medially and compressed (**arrows**). No neoplasm is visible.

B, aortogram, showing a highly vascular neoplasm to the left of the aorta and just above the origin of the superior mesenteric artery. This is in the region of the organ of Zuckerkandl (**a**). It appears to derive its blood supply from two lumbar arteries (**b**). This is an early roentgenogram demonstrating the arteries.

C, later roentgenogram of the same injection. The tumor blush (**arrows**) resulting from filling of arterioles, capillaries and venules is now demonstrated.

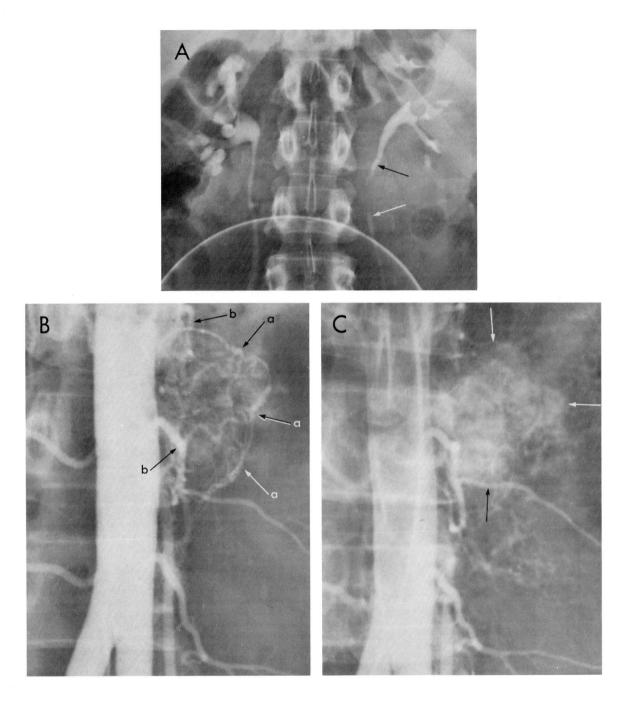

Figure 87 · Pheochromocytoma in Organ of Zuckerkandl / 231

Figure 88.—Extra-adrenal pheochromocytoma arising from the organ of Zuckerkandl.

A, aortogram of a patient with a pheochromocytoma arising from the organ of Zuckerkandl (**a**). This early arterial phase demonstrates vessels arising mainly from three left lumbar arteries passing the periphery of the tumor (**b**) and giving off smaller feeding branches. The tumor displaces the ureter laterally.

B, later exposure, showing the numerous small vessels supplying the tumor (**c**). The lumbar arteries are also demonstrated (**b**).

Pheochromocytomas in this region are difficult to identify by pneumography. They may deviate the ureters, as in Figures 87, *A*, and 88, *A*, but are best demonstrated by arteriography.

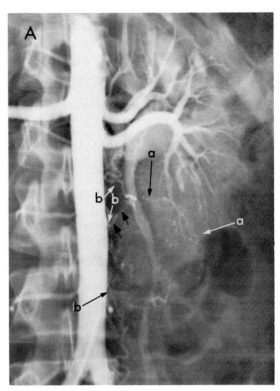

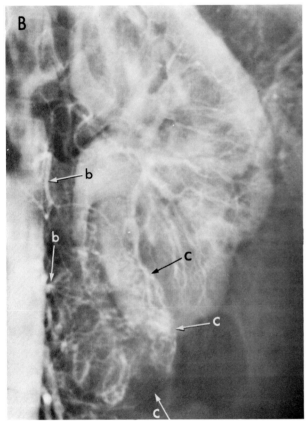

Figure 88 · Pheochromocytoma in Organ of Zuckerkandl / 233

Figure 89.—Metastases from pheochromocytoma.

Posteroanterior chest roentgenogram, showing numerous metastatic growths in the mediastinum (**a**) and both sides of the chest (**b**). Many of the lesions in the right side of the thorax are probably of pleural origin. The anterior portion of the right fourth rib has been destroyed (**c**).

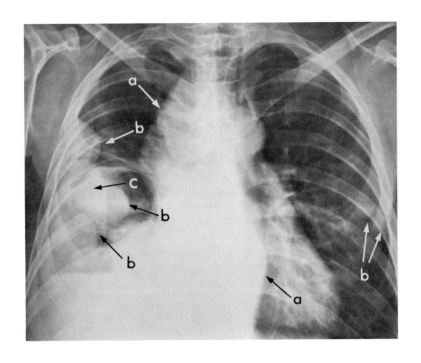

Figure 89 · Pheochromocytoma: Metastases / 235

PART 6

The Ovaries

Ovarian Neoplasms

IN NO ORGAN in the body does as wide a variety of cysts and neoplasms originate as in the ovary. The numerous classifications of ovarian tumors presented by various authors are an indication of the complexity of the subject. To enumerate all the various cysts and tumors of the ovary is beyond the scope of this volume, particularly since their roentgen appearance in most instances is nonspecific. Another volume in this series deals specifically with such tumors.

The following is a brief survey of the more common ovarian cysts and tumors, including those in which a relatively specific diagnosis is sometimes feasible by roentgen examination.

SEROUS CYSTADENOMA AND CYSTADENOCARCINOMA.—Kistner,[1] in a review of 2,181 ovarian neoplasms of all types and stages of malignancy at the Free Hospital for Women, found 620 (24.5%) benign and malignant serous tumors. The benign comprised 65% and the malignant 35%. The malignant serous tumors were nearly three times as common as the malignant mucinous tumors, whereas the ratio of benign serous and mucinous tumors was about 1:1. Serous cystomas are most common between 20 and 50 years, reaching their peak incidence in the third and fourth decades. Malignant serous tumors are more common in patients between 40 and 60 years.

Pathologic changes.—Both benign and malignant forms may be bilateral (20–50%), and generally both are large spherical cysts that vary in diameter up to 40 cm but may be as small as 1–2 cm. Allan and Hertig[2] reported that 56% in their series of serous cystadenocarcinomas were larger than 15 cm in diameter, 40% were 5–15 cm, and only 3–9% were smaller than 5 cm. The benign forms were generally of smaller size, between 5 and 10 cm diameter. Although the smaller cysts may be unilocular, a tendency to multi-loculation and development of papillary projections is noted in the larger tumors. Typical psammoma bodies are often found in the stroma of these tumors; their significance is unknown. The serous tumors present a spectrum ranging from those that are clearly benign to those with unmistakable malignant characteristics. Demarcation between benign and malignant lesions is not sharp.

---

[1] Kistner, R. W.: *Gynecology: Principles and Practice* (Chicago: Year Book Medical Publishers, 1964).

[2] Allan, M. S., and Hertig, A. T.: Carcinoma of the ovary, Am. J. Obst. & Gynec. 58:640, October, 1949.

Mucinous cystadenoma and cystadenocarcinoma.—Some authors prefer the term "pseudomucinous" to designate these tumors since the cyst fluid, unlike true mucin, is soluble in water and dilute acids; however, like true mucin, it is precipitated by alcohol.

Although the incidence of benign mucinous cystadenomas is approximately the same as that of the benign serous cystadenomas, the mucinous cystadenocarcinoma is only one-third as common as the serous cystadenocarcinoma. The mucinous cystomas occur more frequently during the third to fifth decades, almost never before puberty and only occasionally after the menopause.

Pathologic changes.—Grossly, the mucinous tumors closely resemble the serous cystomas. Their tendency toward bilaterality is less marked than that of serous tumors, approximately 5% of the benign and 20% of the malignant forms being bilateral.

Both in benign and in malignant form, the mucinous tumors may be large, the size varying from 1 to 50 cm and most measuring 15–30 cm. The largest tumor on record was said to weigh 328 pounds.

The malignant mucinous tumors differ from the serous cystadenocarcinomas in that metastasis from, or rupture of, the former may give rise to pseudomyxoma peritonei.

Cystic teratoma.—Cystic teratomas or dermoids account for 10–15% of all ovarian neoplasms. They may develop at any age but are relatively rare before puberty. The peak incidence is between 20 and 40 years.

Pathologic changes.—Up to 15% of these tumors are bilateral and are relatively small compared to other ovarian neoplasms. Most of them are less than 10 cm in diameter, and only rarely do they exceed 15 cm. The neoplasms originate from the predominantly ectodermal differentiation of totipotential cells. The cysts may be multilocular but more commonly are unilocular. The lining of the cyst is typically epidermal, and the contents may include tangled masses of hair with thick oily fluid, teeth, bone or cartilage. Some 2–3% of teratomas are composed entirely or largely of thyroid tissue (struma ovarii).

Fewer than 1% of teratomatous growths become malignant. In these rare instances, the tumors are ordinarily compact, solid, rapidly growing neoplasms and are usually unilateral.

Non-neoplastic functional cysts.—*Follicular cysts* originate in unruptured graafian follicles or in follicles that have ruptured and immediately sealed. They are so commonplace that they are virtually a physiologic variant. The cysts may be single, but are usually multiple, and rarely exceed 1–1.5 cm in diameter.

The *Stein-Leventhal syndrome* is characterized by the accumulation of many follicle cysts within the ovary. Typically, the patient is in the late teens or early twenties when menstrual irregularity or amenorrhea, obesity, hirsutism and sterility may be noted. On physical examination, enlarged polycystic ovaries are apparent which at surgery are symmetrical and may be three to four times normal size. The cut section demonstrates multiple follicle cysts enclosed by a thick fibrous capsule.

Corpus luteum cysts occur less often than do follicle cysts and tend to be slightly larger, up to 2–3 cm in diameter.

In ordinary conditions, the non-neoplastic cysts are of little clinical significance, and only occasionally do they reach sufficient size to be recognized roentgenographically. Larger cysts are of importance clinically in that they may resemble neoplastic masses. In these instances, generally, the roentgen examination is of no value in excluding the diagnosis of true neoplasm.

FIBROMA.—Fibromas are relatively common and account for about 10% of all ovarian neoplasms. About 10% are bilateral.

Pathologic changes.—The tumors average 6 cm in size and are dense, usually hard, fibrous tumors. Ascites is found in about 40% of the patients in whom the tumors measure more than 6 cm in diameter. The ascites is usually ascribed either to pronounced venous stasis within these tumors or to increased transudation through greatly dilated lymphatics. Occasionally, with the ascites, pleural effusion may be associated, usually on the right side. The combination of ovarian tumor, ascites and pleural effusion has been designated Meigs' syndrome.

GRANULOSA-THECA CELL TUMORS.—These are tumors composed of various elements of the graafian follicle. At one time, these neoplasms were separated into granulosa cell tumors, theca cell tumors and luteomas, on the basis of the resemblance of the tumor cell to the cell forms in the graafian follicle and corpus luteum. This separation has since been dropped because of the many mixtures of cell types present in these tumors.

Robbins[3] indicated that these tumors account for perhaps fewer than 9% of all ovarian tumors. Tumors of this variety may occur at from 1 to 90 years of age. Most granulosa cell tumors, however, develop during the postmenopausal years and only a few in the prepubertal period.

Pathologic changes.—The tumors vary in size from microscopic foci to large, encapsulated masses up to 40 cm in diameter. A correlation between the age of the patient, size of the tumor and duration of symptoms is not apparent. The granulosa cell tumors are usually unilateral, but as many as 12% of them may be bilateral. Thecomas are almost always unilateral. The

---

[3] Robbins, S. L.: *Pathology* (3rd ed.; Philadelphia: W. B. Saunders Company, 1967).

major clinical significance of these tumors arises from their elaboration of estrogens. The most common symptom of the granulosa-theca cell tumors is uterine bleeding in up to 75% of patients. The abnormal bleeding may be a reflection of endometrial carcinoma, found in 15–25% of patients with granulosa cell tumor. In the prepubertal patient, signs of precocious puberty may be apparent.

ARRHENOBLASTOMA.—The arrhenoblastoma is extremely rare and is of interest primarily because of its masculinizing effects. Only a few hundred cases have been reported. The tumor is present chiefly in young women of child-bearing age and is unilateral in 95% of the cases.

Pathologic changes.—The average size of the arrhenoblastoma is 12–14 cm, but it may vary from microscopic size to 28 cm. The tumor is usually smooth but may be lobulated. About 20% of these tumors recur or metastasize.

Clinically, the tumor is characteristically associated with amenorrhea, defeminization and virilization as a result of excessive androgen secretion. An extremely rare tumor, the *gynandroblastoma,* is composed of a mixture of morphologic elements compatible with both granulosa cell tumor and arrhenoblastoma. These may produce both masculinizing and feminizing hormones.

ROENTGEN FEATURES OF OVARIAN TUMORS

With a few exceptions, roentgen examination of patients with ovarian tumors does not permit a definite diagnosis. Typical changes in a patient with clinical evidence of an ovarian mass include: a pelvic soft tissue mass; obstruction or deviation, or both, of one or both ureters on excretory urography (Figs. 90, 101 and 102), and impression or deviation of the sigmoid colon or small bowel on barium examination (Fig. 98). Thus merely the presence of an ovarian mass is confirmed. That the mass is malignant may be suggested at times by invasion and destruction of the bony pelvis or by fixation and infiltration of bowel (Figs. 96 and 97) or bladder wall, mucosal destruction and, perhaps, fixed filling defects. The differentiation between ovarian masses and uterine masses, such as leiomyomas, endometrial carcinoma and hydatid moles, may be difficult or impossible by roentgenographic means.

Dermoid cysts may present diagnostic changes on roentgenographic examination. Calcification in the cyst wall or in the form of teeth or bone is often visible (Figs. 92–94). The high lipid content in some dermoids may permit their demonstration as a cystic area of diminished density (Fig. 92, *B*).

Any psammous calcification in the region of an ovary on roentgen examination may be accepted as strong evidence of serous cystoma, either benign or malignant (Fig. 95). Occasionally these calcifications are bilateral (Fig. 99).

Pelvic pneumography has been advocated as a means of roentgenographic demonstration of normal and abnormal pelvic structures (Fig. 90, *B*). The procedure is especially useful in instances of equivocal findings on physical examination, obesity, pelvic tenderness or virginal introitus. In patients with the Stein-Leventhal syndrome, a bilateral symmetrical ovarian enlargement may be demonstrated by pelvic pneumography (Fig. 91).

Borell and Fernström[4] reported that arteriography may be of value in distinguishing uterine fibroids from ovarian tumors. In their experience, fibroids are highly vascular lesions whose blood supply is derived from the intramural branches of the uterine artery. Conversely, vascularity of ovarian tumors is sparse and the adnexal branches of the uterine artery are its source of supply.

---

[4] Borell, U., and Fernström, I.: Uterine Arteriography, in Abrams, H. L. (ed.): *Angiography* (Boston: Little, Brown and Company, 1961), Vol. 2.

Figure 90.—Ovarian cysts.

A, excretory urogram: The distal right ureter (**arrows**) is displaced laterally, and the urinary bladder (**a**) is indented from above by an ovarian mass. Diagnosis was follicle cyst of the ovary.

B, pelvic pneumogram: A large ovarian mass (**b**) occupies the right hemipelvis, displacing an enlarged, myomatous uterus (**c**) and normal left ovary (**d**) to the left. This was a corpus luteum cyst.

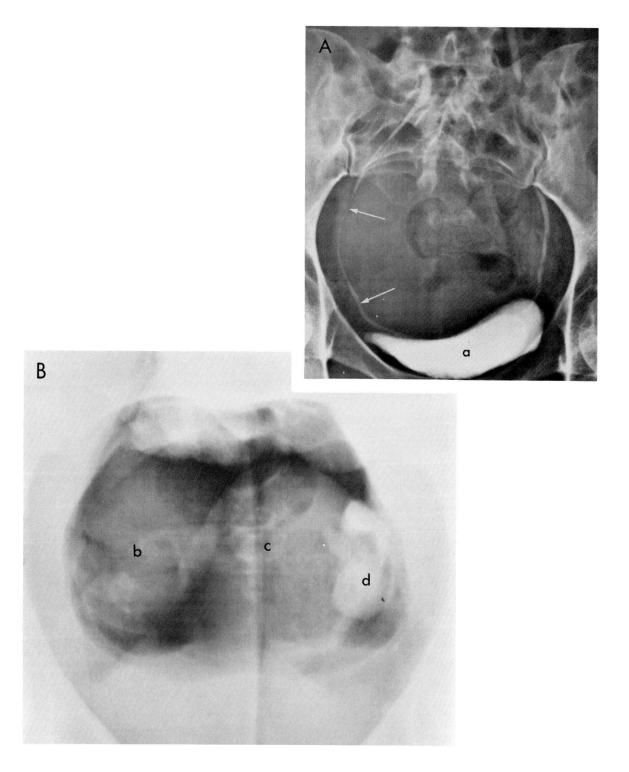

Figure 90 · Ovarian Cysts / 245

Figure 91.—Stein-Leventhal syndrome.

Pelvic pneumogram: Polycystic ovaries are seen as large bilateral ovarian masses (**a**). Bladder (**b**) and uterus (**c**) are normal.

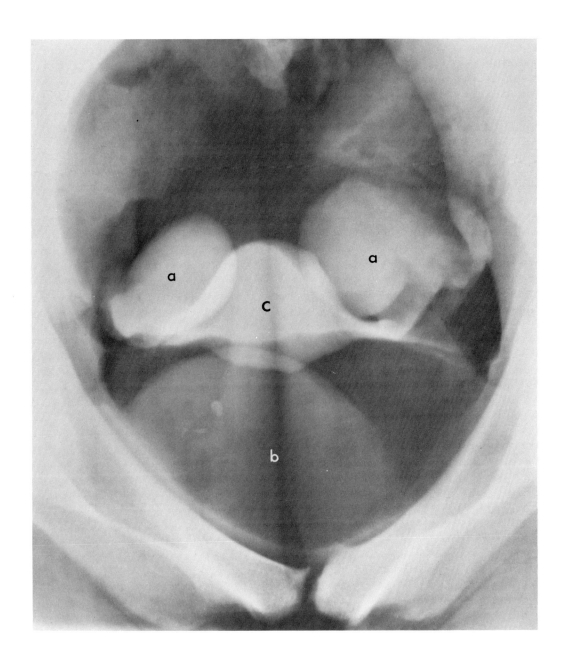

Figure 91 · Stein-Leventhal Syndrome / 247

Figure 92.—Dermoid cysts.

A, anteroposterior view of the pelvis: There is a spherical mass predominantly on the left side of the pelvis, with curvilinear calcification in its wall (**arrows**). A tooth (**a**) and a rudimentary bone (**b**) are contained by the cyst.

B, anteroposterior view of the pelvis: Dermoid cyst of the ovary contains multiple teeth. The zone of diminished density (**arrows**) is a reflection of the high lipid content of the cyst fluid.

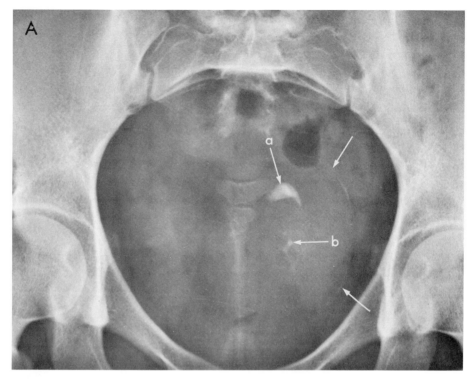

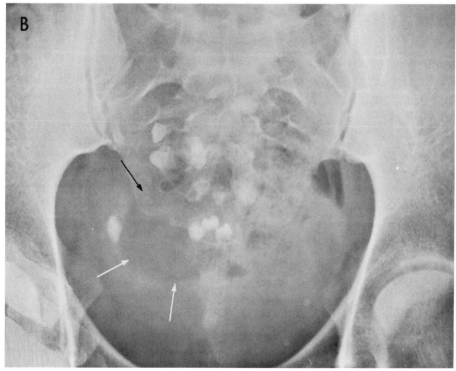

Figure 92 · Dermoid Cysts of the Ovary / 249

Figure 93.—Dermoid cyst of the ovary during pregnancy.

Anteroposterior view of the abdomen: Dermoid cyst of the ovary (**a**) containing three teeth and a rudimentary bone (**b**), displaced out of the pelvis by a pregnant uterus (**arrows**).

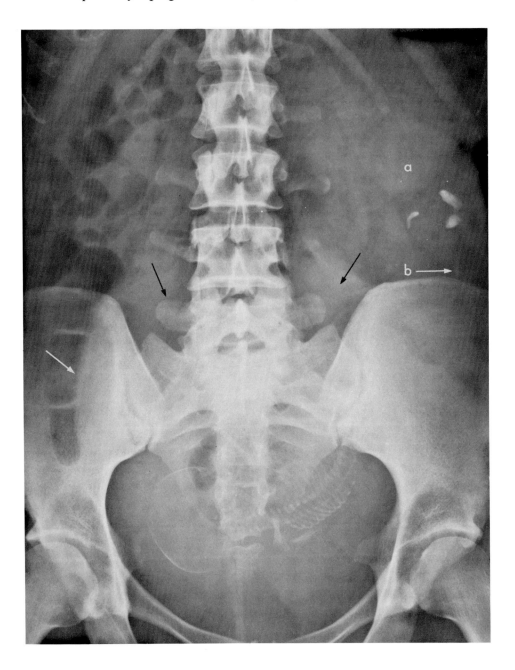

Figure 94.—Teratoma of the ovary.

Excretory urogram: A huge ovarian teratoma with curvilinear calcification in its wall (**arrows**) and containing teeth (**a**), bone (**b**) and amorphous calcification (**c**).

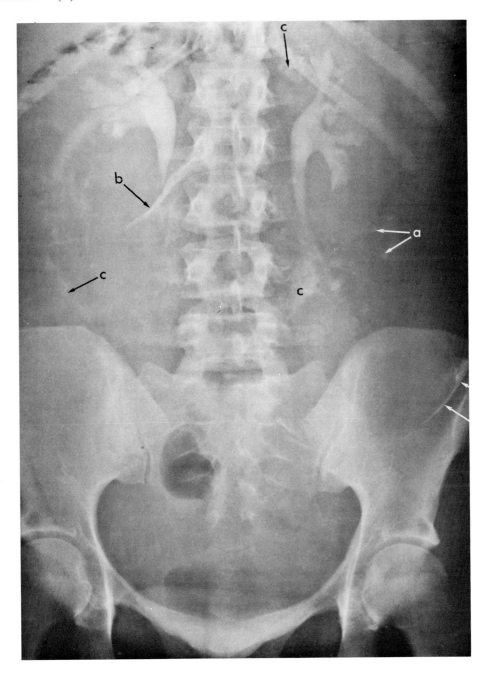

Figure 94 · Teratoma / 251

Figure 95.—Serous cystadenocarcinoma.

Anteroposterior view of the pelvis: A round mass in the right hemipelvis, with calcification in its wall (**arrows**). Histologic examination revealed that the calcification was in the cyst wall and was of the psammous type.

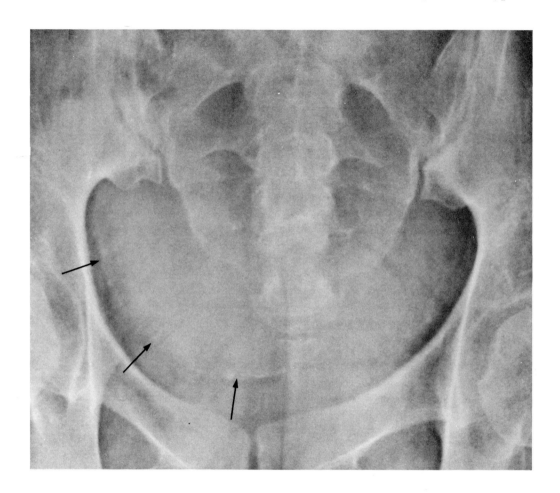

Figure 96.—Ovarian papillary carcinoma involving the sigmoid.

Barium enema examination: Large nodular defects (**arrows**) are present within the barium-filled sigmoid which represent serosal implants with mucosal infiltration by a papillary carcinoma of the ovary.

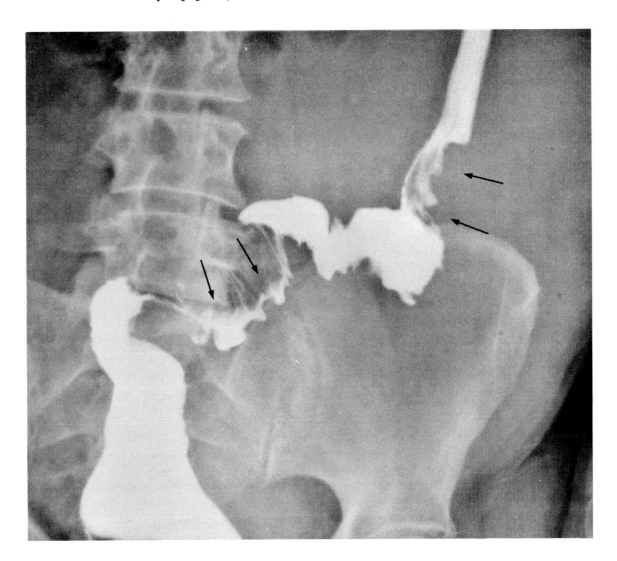

Figure 96 · Ovarian Carcinoma Involving Sigmoid / 253

Figure 97.—Serous cystadenocarcinoma involving the colon.

Barium enema examination: Barium has entered a large spherical cavity (**arrows**) which communicates with the rectosigmoid colon. A serous cystadenocarcinoma of the ovary had eroded through the colonic wall to rupture into the lumen of the large bowel.

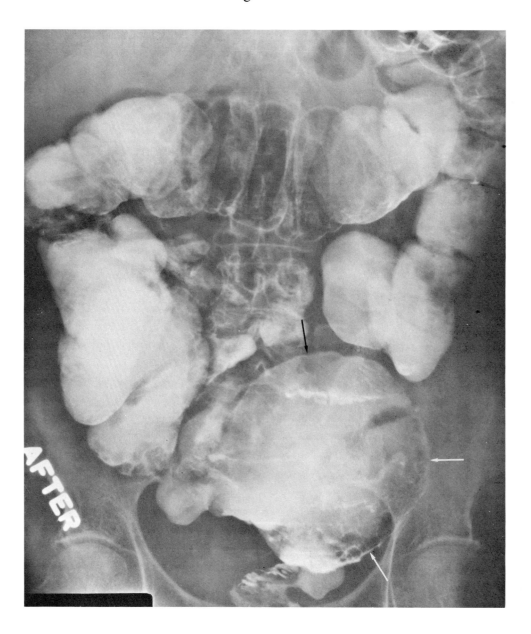

Figure 98.—Carcinoma of the ovary involving the colon.

Barium enema examination: A nodular defect is present along the wall of the sigmoid colon (**arrows**). In addition to the smooth extrinsic pressure defect, there is alteration of the colonic mucosa, as demonstrated by thickening or edema of the mucosal folds. Diagnosis was carcinoma of the ovary metastatic to the mesocolon and wall of the sigmoid colon.

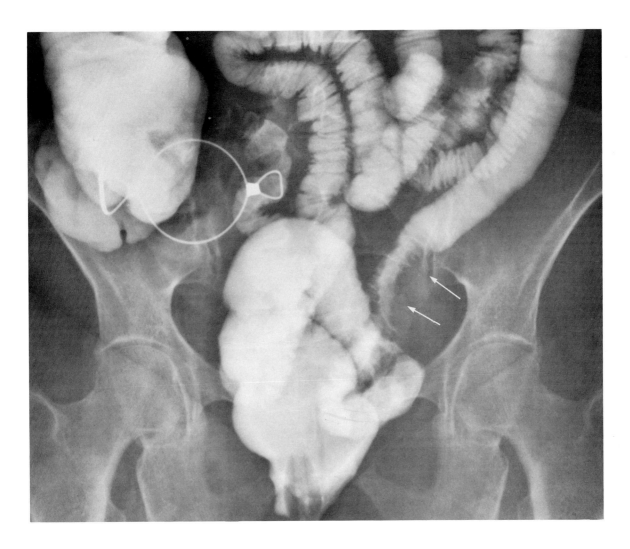

Figure 98 · Colon Metastases from Ovarian Carcinoma / 255

Figure 99.—Bilateral ovarian serous cystadenoma.

Anteroposterior view of the pelvis: Demonstrating bilateral serous cystadenomas (**a**) containing psammous calcifications. The residual barium within the rectum (**x**) is from the prior gastrointestinal examination.

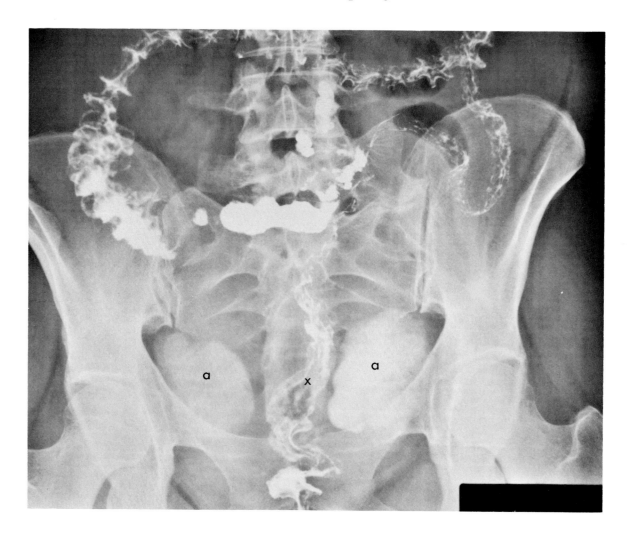

Figure 100.—Dysgerminoma.

Anteroposterior view of the abdomen: Dysgerminoma (**arrows**) of the ovary outlined by air introduced into the peritoneal cavity. The huge tumor has grown out of the pelvis into the abdomen.

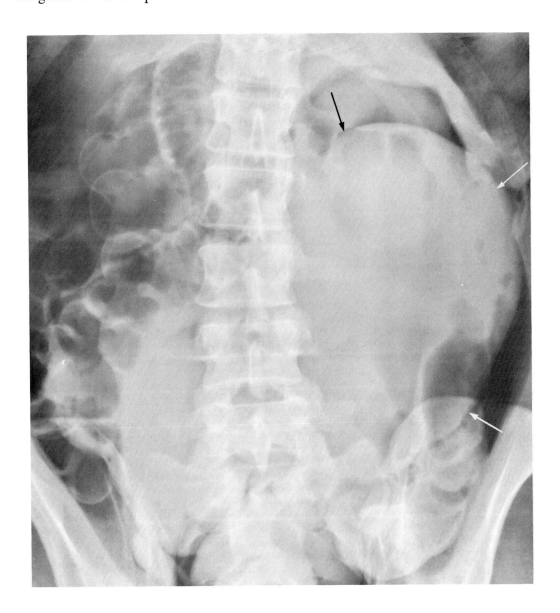

Figure 100 · **Dysgerminoma** / **257**

Figure 101.—Granulosa cell tumor of the ovary.

Excretory urogram: Demonstrating nonfunction of the hydronephrotic left kidney (**arrows**) secondary to long-standing obstruction. The collecting structures of the right kidney (**a**) are slightly dilated. The distal ureter (**b**) is compressed and displaced lateraliy by the ovarian mass, which also causes extrinsic compression of the bladder (**c**).

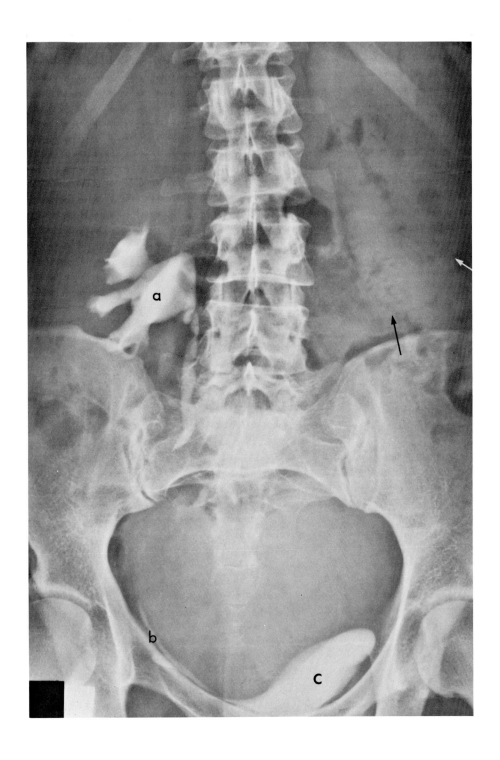

Figure 101 · Granulosa Cell Tumor / 259

Figure 102.—Meigs' syndrome.

A, posteroanterior view of the chest of a woman with an ovarian fibroma. The costophrenic sulcus on the right is obliterated by pleural fluid (**arrows**).

B (same patient as in *A*). A hazy density over the entire abdomen reflects the presence of ascites. Both distal ureters are displaced laterally by an ovarian fibroma (**arrows**) which also impresses the bladder from above (**a**).

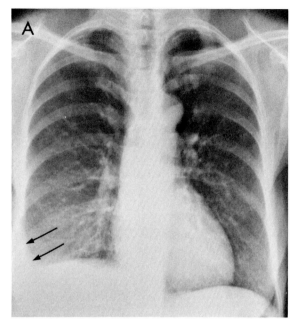

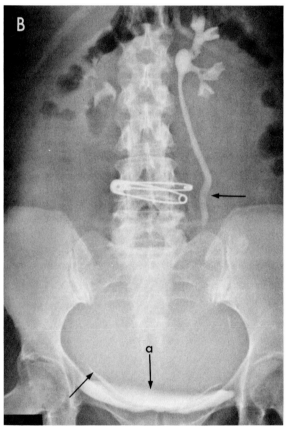

Figure 102 · Meigs' Syndrome / 261

PART 7

The Testes

Tumors of the Testis

PATHOLOGY.—Dixon and Moore[1] have divided testicular tumors into two general categories: tumors of germ cell origin, constituting 96.5% of testicular tumors, and the nongerminal tumors, constituting 3.5%. Of the *germinal tumors,* four principal histologic patterns have been defined: seminoma, embryonal carcinoma, teratoma, and choriocarcinoma. Seminoma is the most frequent of the germinal tumors, comprising approximately 41%, and tends to occur in an older age group. These tumors are composed of large round or polygonal cells, quite uniform in size, with clear cytoplasm. Grossly, the involved testis may be slightly or greatly enlarged but usually maintains its normal contour, due to the fact that the surrounding tunica is seldom invaded.

Embryonal carcinoma, teratoma and choriocarcinoma are closely related tumors, having in common their origin from totipotential cells. Grossly, embryonal carcinomas represent about 30% of germinal tumors and are among the smallest testicular tumors. The contour of the testis is distorted more often than in the case of seminoma because these tumors frequently invade the tunica and extend into surrounding structures, particularly the epididymis and cord. Microscopically, the pattern of growth may vary from the highly undifferentiated form, in which large sheets or masses of anaplastic cells are created, to more well-differentiated forms with well-developed glandular patterns. Many of these tumors grow as almost pure adenocarcinomas.[2]

Teratomas and teratocarcinomas are relatively common, ranking between seminoma and embryonal carcinoma in frequency. These tumors demonstrate areas of organoid differentiation which resemble normal adult tissues. Structures such as cartilage, muscle and clusters of squamous epithelium are most often found, although occasionally such tissues as thyroid, bronchial epithelium, brain and bone may be encountered. Metastases may occur even when no histologic areas of malignancy are observed. Malignant behavior is more likely when these tumors occur in young adults than in children.

Choriocarcinomas comprise only 1% of the germinal tumors of the testis but are the most malignant lesions of the group.[3] They are usually small,

[1] Dixon, F. J., and Moore, R. A.: Tumors of the Male Sex Organs, Sect. VII, Fasc. 31b and 32, of Armed Forces Institute of Pathology *Atlas of Tumor Pathology* (Washington, D.C.: 1952).
[2] Robbins, S. L.: *Pathology* (3rd ed.; Philadelphia: W. B. Saunders Company, 1967).
[3] Anderson, W. A. D.: *Pathology* (5th ed.; St. Louis: C. V. Mosby Company, 1966).

frequently hemorrhagic and necrotic lesions consisting of cytotrophoblastic and syncytiotrophoblastic cells arranged in papillae or villi.

Nongerminal tumors of the testis are relatively uncommon, comprising less than 4% of testicular tumors. Although such nongerminal tumors as neurofibromas, angiomas and fibromas occur, only two nongerminal tumors are of exclusively gonadal origin: the interstitial cell tumor, and the andro-blastoma. Approximately one third of the interstitial cell tumors occur in children. These tumors are associated with clinical evidence of precocious puberty caused by excessive androgen secretion. In adults, signs and symp-toms resulting from androgen hypersecretion are relatively uncommon. Gynecomastia is a common finding but is not well explained. Interstitial cell tumors are small, usually spherical lesions derived from the cells of Leydig. Less than 10% exhibit malignant behavior.

Androblastoma is the homologue of the ovarian arrhenoblastoma and may be associated with feminization of the male. Grossly, the tumors are moderately large lesions which enlarge but do not distort the contour of the testis. Histologically, three types of androblastoma have been defined: stro-mal, tubular, and mixed stromal and tubular. None of the reported andro-blastomas have been malignant.

CLINICAL COURSE.—The clinical course of all of the testicular tumors is similar in many respects. Often, enlargement or palpable hardness of the affected testis is noted as the first symptom. Crytorchidism appears to be a predisposing factor to the development of malignancy. An 11- to 40-fold increase in the incidence of malignancy has been reported in association with maldescent of the testes.

Most metastases from testicular tumors occur by way of the lymphatics, although choriocarcinomas spread predominantly through the blood stream, and vascular spread is possible in any case of testicular carcinoma. On the right side, the primary lymph nodes are just inferior to the junction of the spermatic vein and the vena cava. On the left, the primary nodes are in the para-aortic region around the level of the renal vein. Sites of metastasis include, in decreasing frequency, the primary lymph nodes, lungs, inguinal nodes and spermatic cord. Less commonly, the mediastinum, liver, adrenals, kidney, pancreas, brain and bones may be involved.[4]

RADIOGRAPHIC FINDINGS.—Although roentgenology has little to offer in the diagnosis of primary testicular tumors, roentgen examination may play an important role in the assessment of metastatic disease.

Large retroperitoneal masses may displace various portions of the barium-filled gut (Figs. 103–105). In the chest, mediastinal or hilar lymph node

---

[4] Murphy, W. T.: *Pathology* (3rd ed.; Philadelphia: W. B. Saunders Company, 1967).

enlargement, or both, is frequently demonstrable roentgenographically. Hematogenous spread of testicular tumors is often manifested by the appearance of multiple, although occasionally single, well-demarcated, spherical pulmonary masses (Fig. 106).

Excretory urography may at times demonstrate displacement of one or both kidneys and ureters by large nodes involved by metastatic tumor (Figs. 107 and 111). Displacement or distortion of the inferior vena cava (Fig. 108), particularly in cases of right-sided tumors, is often demonstrable by inferior venacavography. Arteriography too may reveal significant vascular distortions and displacements (Fig. 109).

Lymphangiography has played an increasingly prominent role in the assessment of retroperitoneal nodal involvement by testicular tumors as well as by the lymphomas (Fig. 107). Routine foot lymphangiography may demonstrate displacement of normal lymphatic chains, obstruction of the lymphatic flow and collateral lymphatic flow (Fig. 110). Cook *et al.*[5] have demonstrated tumor in the primary lymph nodes draining the testes by injecting contrast material directly into lymphatics of the spermatic cord. These nodes are not filled by routine foot lymphangiography.

Skeletal metastases (Fig. 111) of testicular tumors have been documented by Sum *et al.*[6] In their series, skeletal metastases were found on biopsy or at autopsy in 10 of 167 patients with testicular tumors. Osteolytic metastases were demonstrated roentgenologically in 5 patients and osteoblastic metastases in 2. In both of the latter, the primary tumor was seminoma.

[5] Cook, F. E., *et al.*: Testicular carcinoma and lymphangiography, Radiology: 420, March, 1965.

[6] Sum, P. W.; Roswit, B., and Unger, S. M.: Skeletal metastases from malignant testicular tumors: A report of 10 cases with osteolytic and osteoblastic changes, Am. J. Roentgenol. 83:704, April, 1960.

Figure 103.—Seminoma testis metastases.

A, posteroanterior roentgenogram, showing the stomach (**a**) and duodenum (**b**) displaced laterally and partial obstruction (**c**).

B (same patient as in *A*), right lateral roentgenogram, showing the stomach (**a**) and duodenum (**b**) displaced forward.

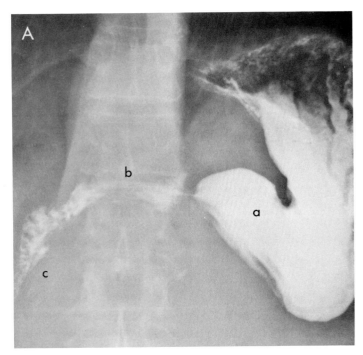

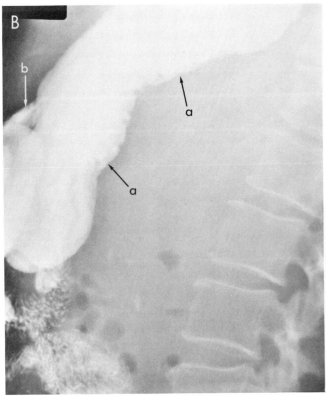

Figure 103 · Seminoma Testis: Metastases / 269

Figure 104.—Mixed choriocarcinoma and teratocarcinoma with metastases.

A, anteroposterior roentgenogram of a gastrointestinal series: Displacement of the lesser curvature of the stomach to the left (**arrows**). The tumor has spread extensively in the retroperitoneal space, particularly on the left side. The proximal (**a**) and distal (**b**) duodenum are flattened by pressure of the tumor.

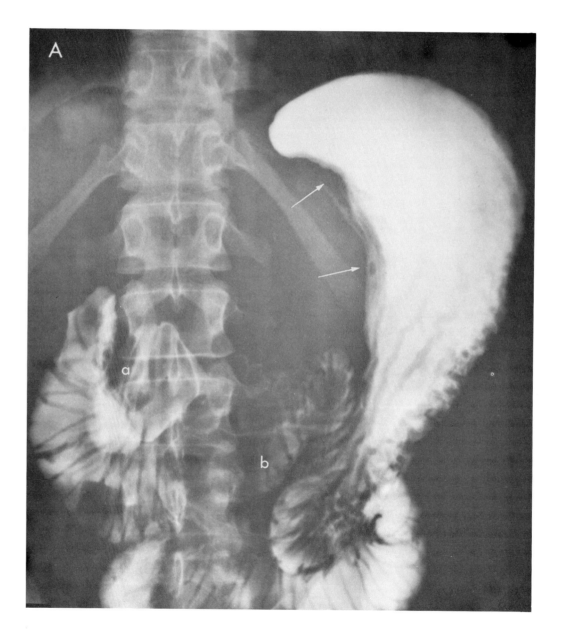

B (same patient as in *A*), left lateral view: Displacement of the posterior portion of the stomach by a lobulated retroperitoneal mass (**arrows**).

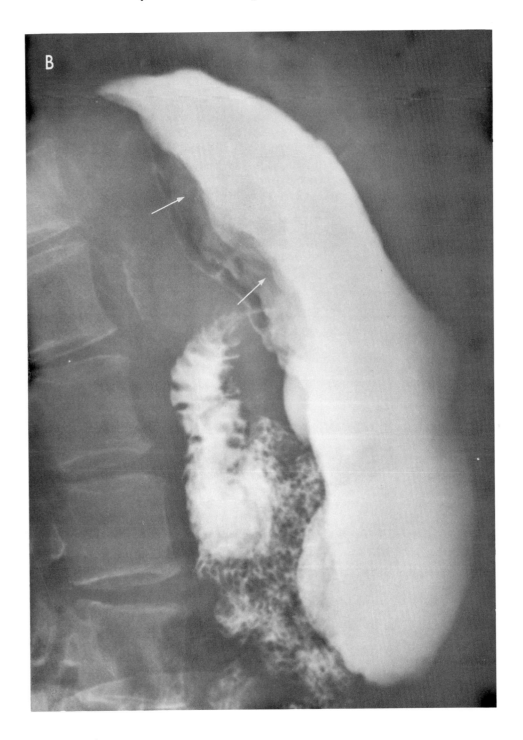

Figure 104 · Mixed Choriocarcinoma and Teratocarcinoma / 271

Figure 105.—Embryonal cell carcinoma with metastases.

A, anteroposterior view after barium enema: A metastatic tumor that has surrounded and compressed the rectum and rectosigmoid (**arrows**). The mucosa of the rectum has not been destroyed.

B (same patient as in *A*), lateral roentgenogram of the rectum: A retroperitoneal mass encircles the rectum but has not destroyed the mucosa. The rectum and sigmoid are constricted (**arrows**). The tumor has increased the space between rectum and sacrum (**a**).

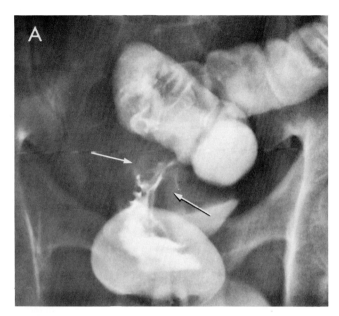

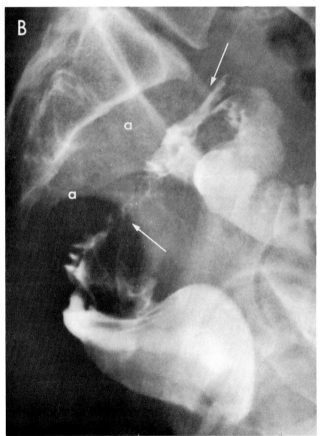

Figure 105 · Embryonal Cell Carcinoma: Metastases / 273

Figure 106.—Choriocarcinoma with metastases.

A, anteroposterior roentgenogram, demonstrating numerous metastatic lesions of various sizes. The larger are more sharply demarcated than the smaller ones. Metastases are predominantly in the lower part of the lungs. These lesions have arisen from hematogenous spread, which is relatively common with choriocarcinoma. The right hilus (a) is greatly enlarged by metastases in the lymph nodes.

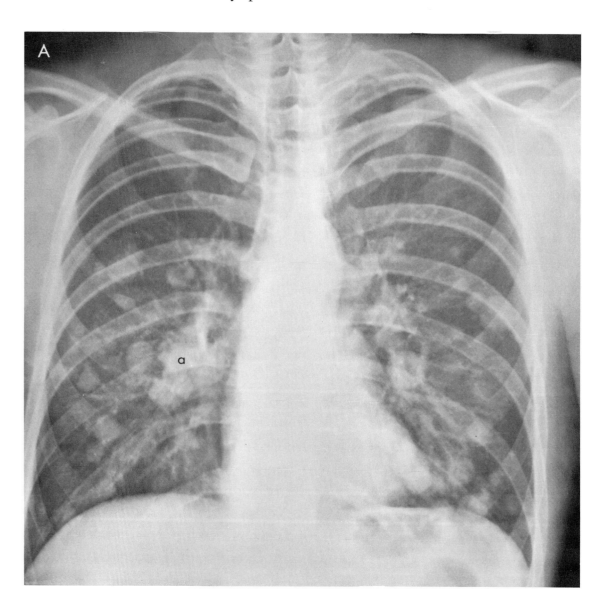

B, intravenous urogram of same patient as in *A*. The left kidney is displaced laterally and rotated, and is appreciably larger than the right, possibly as a result of compression of the renal vein by enlarged lymph nodes. The left ureter is displaced and lobulated due to the retroperitoneal metastases (**arrows**). Contrast material (**x**) remains in some lymph nodes from previous lymphangiography.

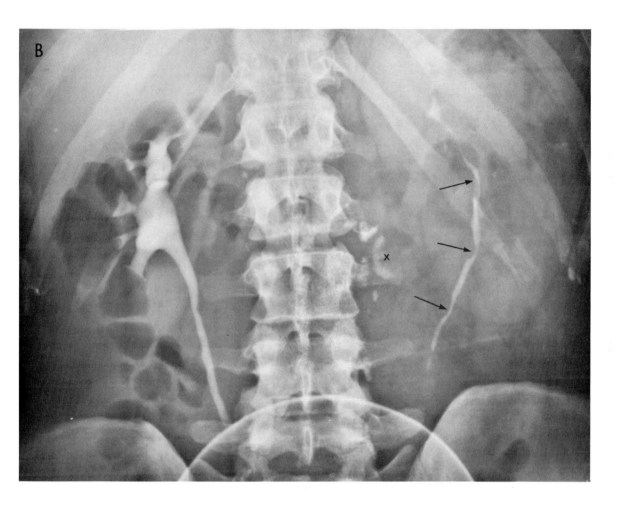

Figure 106 · Choriocarcinoma: Metastases / 275

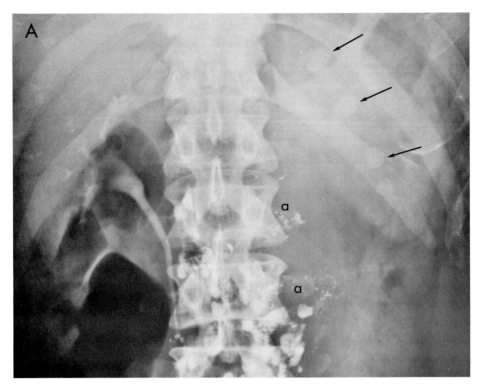

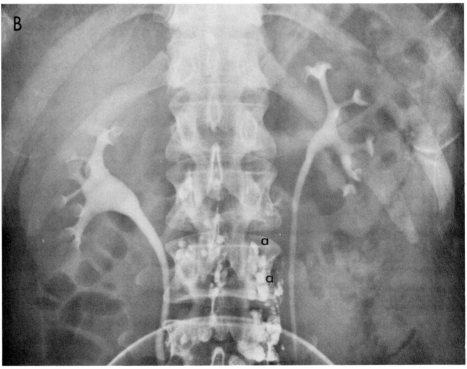

Figure 107.—Embryonal cell carcinoma with retroperitoneal metastases (all
figures from same patient).

A, intravenous urogram obtained 30 minutes after intravenous injection
of contrast material. The right kidney appears to be normal. The left kidney
is displaced upward and laterally, and its calyces are dilated due to partial
obstruction of the kidney pelvis by tumor (**arrows**). Opaque material from
previous lymphangiography outlines enlarged lymph nodes to the left of the
spine (**a**). About one third of left-sided testicular tumors metastasize along
the spermatic lymphatic system and congregate in the spermatic nodes just
below the left renal vein, as in this case.

B, one year later, following radiation therapy, the left kidney is no longer
obstructed and appears to be normal. The enlarged lymph nodes seen in *A*
have decreased remarkably in size (**a**).

C, nine months later, the left kidney is displaced down and laterally, with
an acute angle formed at the ureteropelvic junction (**arrow**). The ureter
draining the right kidney is also displaced by neoplasm (**b**). The lymph
nodes (**a**) appear to be even smaller now than they were in *B*.

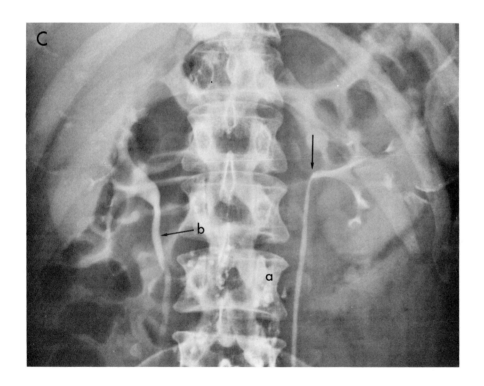

Figure 107 · Embryonal Cell Carcinoma: Metastases / 277

Figure 108.—Seminoma testis with retroperitoneal metastases.

A, venacavogram, anteroposterior view of the inferior vena cava (**a**) following injection of contrast material into the femoral veins. The vena cava is displaced to the right and compressed (**arrows**). Because of compression, there is unusually good filling of the paravertebral venous plexus and ascending lumbar veins (**b**).

B, venacavogram (same patient as in *A*), lateral view. The vena cava is displaced forward by the retroperitoneal mass (**arrows**). Lumbar vertebral bodies are seen faintly at **x**.

(*Continued* in Figure 109.)

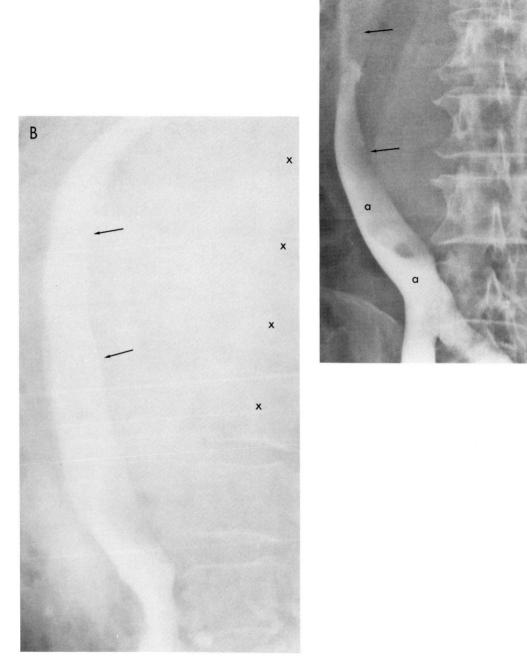

Figure 108 · Seminoma Testis: Metastases / 279

Figure 109.—Seminoma testis with retroperitoneal metastases (same patient as in Figure 108).

A, arteriogram, anteroposterior view, showing the aorta (**a**) and its branches. The superior mesenteric artery gives off intestinal and colic branches (**arrows**), which are stretched. The small vessels are displaced peripherally (**b**). The right renal artery (**c**) is stretched due to lateral displacement of the right kidney by the retroperitoneal mass.

B, arteriogram, late arterial phase. At this time, the stretching and displacement of the branches of the superior mesenteric artery by the retroperitoneal mass is even more noteworthy than in *A*. Arteries affected are: **d,** middle colic; **e,** jejunal branches; **f,** ileocolic; **g,** ileal; **h,** hepatic. Note displacement of the right renal calyces (**x**).

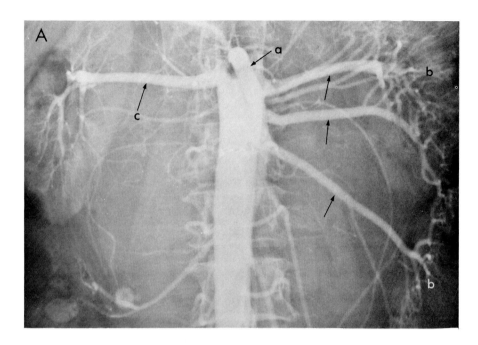

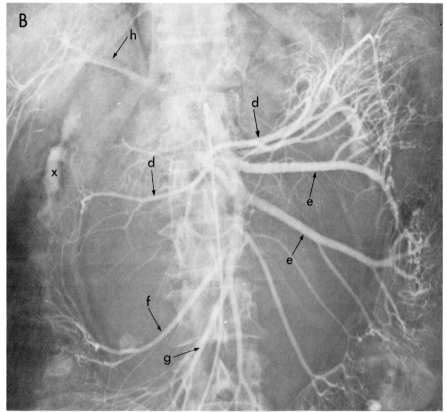

Figure 109 · Seminoma Testis: Metastases / 281

Figure 110.—Embryonal carcinoma and seminoma testis with lymph node invasion.

A, left posterior oblique roentgenogram obtained after lymphangiography performed by injecting contrast material into the lymphatics of the feet of a patient with embryonal carcinoma of the left testis. Large lymph nodes (**a**) with no contrast in their centers indicate the presence of metastatic deposits. These are the para-aortic nodes adjacent to the left renal vein, a typical site of metastases from left-sided testicular tumors.

B, left posterior oblique roentgenogram obtained 24 hours after lymphangiography in a patient with left-sided seminoma testis. A large metastatic tumor (**arrows**) is eccentrically situated in a left para-aortic lymph node. The node is enlarged, and there is no contrast material in the space occupied by the tumor (**a**).

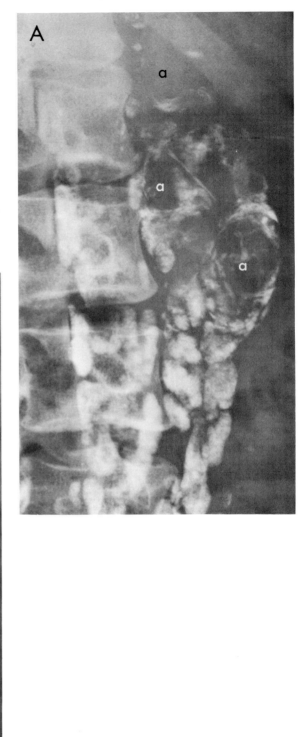

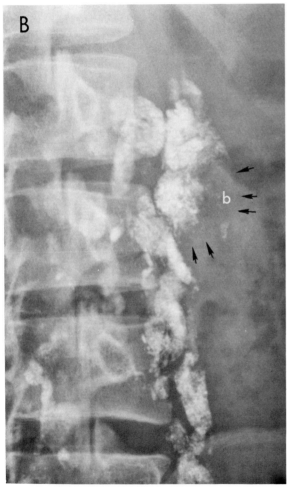

Figure 110 · Testicular Tumors: Lymph Node Invasion / 283

Figure 111.—Leiomyosarcoma of the left testis.

A, intravenous urogram 3 hours after injection of contrast medium. The right kidney of this 3-year-old boy was normal. The dilated calyces, pelvis and ureter of the left kidney were not seen previous to this exposure. The kidney is displaced laterally. The proximal part of the left ureter also is displaced laterally and partially obstructed by the neoplasm (**arrows**), which involved the retroperitoneal lymph nodes and adjacent tissues on the left side.

B (same patient as in *A*), anteroposterior roentgenogram of the right shoulder. There are numerous small irregular destructive lesions of the humerus that produce a mottled appearance (**arrows**). A thin layer of tumor-reactive new bone has been produced by the periosteum medially (**a**).

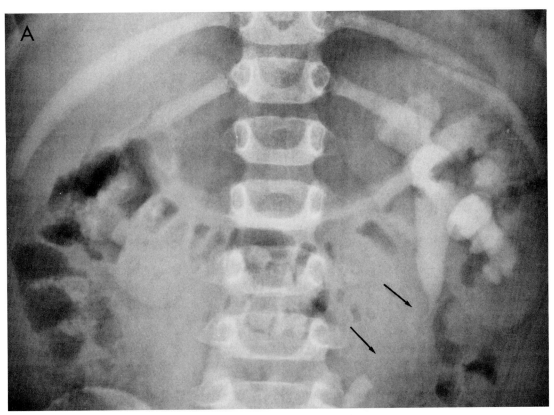

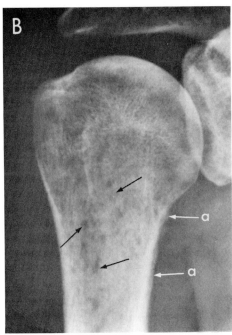

Figure 111 · Leiomyosarcoma with Metastases / 285

PART 8

The Pineal Gland and Hypothalamus

(CEREBRAL TUMORS CAUSING ENDOCRINE DISORDERS)

Tumors of the Pineal Gland

THE FUNCTION of the pineal body has been the subject of past and continuing investigations but remains undecided. The gland has been thought to be involved in somatic growth, endocrine function and sexual development. Pathologic changes include tumors and cysts that encroach on surrounding structures. Indirectly, through encroachment on hypothalamus and aqueduct of Sylvius, or as a result of endocrine secretions by the pineal body, sexual and somatic maturation and growth are accelerated or retarded.

ANATOMY OF THE PINEAL GLAND.—The pineal gland is a midline structure situated above the posterior extremity of the third ventricle. Its base is directed anteriorly, beneath the bulging portion of the corpus callosum, above and behind the posterior white commissure, where it rests on the groove between the quadrigeminal bodies. Laterally, the gland is in relation to the choroid plexus and above, borders on the vein of Galen.

The fully developed pineal gland is composed of masses of cells divided into lobules by connective tissue and vascular septa. The septa enlarge with age. Oval or round pale nuclei appear in the parenchymal cells and are surrounded by stellate or irregular cytoplasm. Small cytoplasmic granules are present after 11 years of age, and vesicular, rounded masses or clear areas are often seen in the nuclei. These structures may indicate secretory activity. Neuroglial cells, mainly astrocytes, are scattered throughout the gland. Calcareous concretions appear histologically soon after puberty. They are evident on roentgenograms in about 25% in the second decade of life and their number increases with age. Occasionally, calcification is visible roentgenographically in younger children.[1]

FUNCTION OF THE PINEAL GLAND.—Melatonin, a substance producing contraction of the pigment granules in melanocytes of some species, is produced only by the pineal body. The substance is released into the circulation and is excreted in the urine. In laboratory animals, physiologic effects on the gonads, thyroid, skin, gut and pituitary gland have been attributed to melatonin. Tissues in or near the pineal gland contain glomerulotropin which may enhance the secretion or release of aldosterone by the adrenal cortex. Many other biologically active substances are noted in high concentration in the pineal body, including serotonin, norepinephrine, 5-methoxyindole acetic acid and 5-hydroxyindole acetic acid.

---

[1] Anderson, W. A. D.: *Pathology* (5th ed.; St. Louis: C. V. Mosby Company, 1966), Vol. 2.

Blood flows through the pineal gland rapidly at a rate second only to that of the kidney according to weight.

CLINICAL CHANGES WITH PINEAL TUMORS.—The neurologic signs of importance are caused by increased intracranial pressure resulting from compression of the aqueduct of Sylvius. Headache is followed by blurring of vision, diplopia, Argyll Robertson pupils, papilledema, vomiting, drowsiness and paralysis of extraocular muscles. This paralysis prevents upward gaze, indicative of involvement of the corpora quadrigemina.

In about one third of the boys, but not in girls, with tumors, sexual development is premature. This prematurity has been interpreted as an indication that the pineal body is an endocrine gland that inhibits sexual development in boys. The tumors were believed to destroy the glandular tissue that controls this inhibitory secretion, thus causing precocious sexual development. Other investigators have expressed the belief that a hormone, elaborated by the tumor directly, caused sexual precocity. The alteration of sexual development has also been attributed to invasion or compression of the hypothalamus by the tumor. In 70% of the patients with pineal tumors and precocious sexuality, hypothalamic signs were present. These consisted of diabetes insipidus, polyphagia, obesity, somnolence and abnormal body temperature. Pineal teratomas and cysts, however, also produce the same endocrine symptoms, but in only a few instances of sexual precocity has the diagnosis of parenchymal pinealoma been verified histologically. Much experimental evidence has added support to one theory or another. The effect on sexual maturation by pineal elaboration of hormones has not been satisfactorily resolved, however. The clinical, laboratory and roentgen features associated with premature sexual development are similar to those in males with hypothalamic tumors. These are discussed later.

Primary tumors of the pineal body are rare and consist of pinealoma, gliomatous tumor, teratoma and germinoma, among others. In a series of more than 4,000 tumors of the central nervous system, only 35 pinealomas were found.[2] Pineal tumors of various types may arise in ectopic pinealomas. More than 50% of pineal tumors develop before age 20. These tumors are three times more common in males than in females.

PINEALOMA.—The most frequent tumor of the pineal body is composed of groups of large parenchymal cells that usually reproduce in appearance some stage in development of the organ. The parenchymal cells are separated by smaller darker cells. Some pinealomas invade contiguous tissues extensively or implant in the ventricles or on cranial nerves. These tumors tend

---

[2] Kernohan, J. W., and Sayre, G. P.: Tumors of the Central Nervous System, (Sect. X, Fasc. 35, of Armed Forces Institute of Pathology *Atlas of Tumor Pathology* (Washington, D.C.: 1952).

to be associated with depressed gonadal function. Pinealomas arise from embryonic cell rests in the brain stem, the base of the brain, the optic chiasm or nerves and the hypothalamic-pituitary region. The tumors may be associated with sexual infantilism and other evidence of pituitary failure, as well as with diabetes insipidus. In at least 2 patients with ectopic pinealoma, precocious sexual and somatic development were reported.

Germinomas rarely arise in the pineal body.

GLIOMATOUS TUMORS.—Usually, these tumors are spongioblastomas and ependymomas and probably arise from the neuroglial cells of the pineal body. The ependymomas differ from those found elsewhere in that they contain large pale cells similar to pineal parenchymal cells. Numerous mitotic and giant cells may be present, indicating a high degree of malignancy. With gliomatous and teratomatous tumors, sexual precocity is three times as common as with parenchymal tumors.

TERATOMAS.—This type of tumor is considered common in the pineal region. In some instances it is associated with precocious somatic and sexual development, mainly when the tumor destroys the pineal parenchyma. It is a tumor that contains elements of all three germ layers, which may include epidermis, cartilage, bone, connective tissue, muscle and brain. It does not appear to be malignant usually, but may recur after surgical removal.

ROENTGEN FEATURES

PLAIN ROENTGENOGRAMS OF THE SKULL.—Abnormal calcification is noted on roentgenograms to be associated with about 50% of pineal tumors. An eccentric pineal tumor may displace the normal calcified portion in any direction (Fig. 112). Evidence of normal pineal calcification is not common before 10 years of age, and its presence may indicate a pineal tumor. Extensive calcification over an area larger than the normal pineal gland, at any age, indicates the possibility of a neoplasm (Fig. 113). The calcification of gliomatous pineal tumors is similar to that of gliomas elsewhere and may be punctate, amorphous, trabecular or arborizing. Only a small part of the tumor may be calcified (Figs. 113 and 114). Teratomas and dermoids of the pineal gland are often calcified. Bone and dental structures may then be seen in large lesions. Fat in these tumors may be represented on the roentgenogram as an area of radiolucency with or without associated calcification. Germinomas may calcify.

On roentgenograms, the skull may show evidence of increased intracranial pressure. In young children, the sutures may be wide and the head enlarged. With only slightly elevated pressure or arrested hydrocephalus, the head may be large with normal width of sutures. The coronal and sagittal sutures are most frequently affected. After the age of puberty, widening of the sutures is uncommon. Other evidence of increased pressure includes exaggeration of convolutional markings and enlargement of the occipital and other emissary vein channels. The cranial vault or base may be thin. The interior cortex of the sella turcica, particularly the anterior dorsum sellae and posterior clinoid processes, may be eroded. Eventually, the sella enlarges. With hydrocephalus from pineal tumor, the third ventricle dilates, resulting in erosion of the posterior clinoids, dorsum and tuberculum sellae.

PNEUMOGRAPHY.—Because of signs of increased intracranial pressure, ventriculography is usually performed. Typically, the lateral ventricles and anterior parts of the third ventricle are enlarged (Fig. 113). The tumor obstructs the posterior third ventricle and prevents gas from filling the aqueduct or fourth ventricle (Figs. 112–114). The anterior part of the tumor that projects into the third ventricle is outlined by gas. Small pineal tumors may be diagnosed before complete obstruction of the aqueduct because of obliteration of the suprapineal recess. On frontal roentgenograms, the mass is seen to project into the dilated third ventricle (Fig. 115). Extension along the floor of the third ventricle, a distant metastatic lesion or an ectopic neoplasm may be identified (Figs. 116 and 117). Primary or metastatic tumors in adjacent areas of the brain may simulate pineal neoplasms. Usually, they do not appear as a convex or hemispheric mass that projects into the posterior third ventricle nor do they obliterate the suprapineal recess.

In addition to the above changes, pneumoencephalography may demonstrate obliteration of the quadrigeminal cistern and a narrow, straightened or depressed aqueduct.

Depending on their position, ectopic pineal tumors may produce roentgen signs, but are not usually diagnosed preoperatively (Figs. 116–117). They may invade the floor of the third ventricle, simulating a hypothalamic tumor.

ANGIOGRAPHY.—Vertebral arteriography characteristically demonstrates upward and posterior displacement and increased curvature of the posterior choroidal arteries. The tumor displaces the internal cerebral vein upward and backward, producing an angle between it and the great vein of Galen. The distance between the pineal calcification and the internal cerebral vein is increased. Abnormal vessels that "feed" the tumor may be demonstrated.[3-5]

---

[3] Epstein, B. S.: *Pneumoencephalography and Cerebral Angiography* (Chicago: Year Book Medical Publishers, 1966).

[4] Schmitz, A. L., Haveson, S. B., and Hanna, D.: *Illustrative Cranial Neuroradiology* (Springfield, Ill.: Charles C Thomas, Publisher, 1967).

[5] Taveras, J. M., and Wood, E. H.: Diseases of the Nervous System, in Robbins, L. L. (ed.): *Golden's Diagnostic Roentgenology* (Baltimore: Williams & Wilkins Company, 1968), Vol. 1, pp. 1.1–1.943.

Hypothalamic Lesions

Many lesions of the brain may cause endocrine disorders, some by encroaching on or destroying the pituitary gland or infundibulum. The endocrine abnormalities may arise from (*a*) stimulation or inhibition of the secretory activities of the adenohypophysis, (*b*) alteration of the secretory function of the neurohypophysis (diabetes insipidus), or (*c*) direct action on peripheral organs through the autonomic system.

ANATOMY OF THE HYPOTHALAMUS.—The hypothalamus forms the floor and lower lateral walls of the third ventricle. It is bounded anteriorly by the lamina terminalis, which forms the anterior wall of the third ventricle and extends posteriorly to include the mammillary bodies. The hypothalamus is separated from the thalamus, which forms the upper portion of the wall of the ventricle, by a shallow groove called the sulcus hypothalamus.[6] At the anterior inferior border are the optic chiasm and optic tracts, and at the posterior border are the posterior perforated substance and cerebal peduncles.

Four groups of nuclei are of special importance in the consideration of endocrine function:

1. *Anterior group.*—This group includes (*a*) the *supraoptic nucleus*, which lies immediately above the optic chiasm and projects for a short distance along the anterior aspect of the tuber cinereum, and (*b*) the *paraventricular nuclei*, which are a little superior to the supraoptic nucleus in the anterior portion of the wall of the ventricle. The supraoptico-hypophyseal tract of nerve fibers passes from these nuclei to the posterior pituitary body along the infundibular stalk.

2. *Middle group.*—This group of nuclei lies in the floor of the third ventricle just posterior to the infundibulum. It includes the *nucleus tuberalis* and *ventromedial* and *dorsomedial* nuclei.

3. *Lateral group.*—This occupies the lateral part of the tuber cinereum. It includes the *lateral hypothalamic area* and the *lateral tuberal nuclei.*

4. *Posterior group.*—This group includes nuclei that compose the *corpora mammillaria,* two rounded bodies protruding at the base of the brain, and the *posterior hypothalamic nuclei,* which are in the lateral walls of the ventricle just above and anterior to the mammillary bodies.

FUNCTION OF THE HYPOTHALAMUS.—The hypothalamus is a relay center between higher brain regions and the efferent and afferent pathways of the

---

[6] Wilkins, L.: *The Diagnosis and Treatment of Endocrine Disorders in Childhood and Adolescence* (3rd ed.; Springfield, Ill.: Charles C Thomas, Publisher, 1965), p. 454.

sympathetic and parasympathetic centers of the brain stem and spinal cord. It is involved in the regulation of temperature, blood pressure, behavior, emotional response, eating and drinking and the volume and concentration of urine. The endocrine effects are achieved through the elaboration of neurohumeral and hormonal principles. These include vasopressin, oxytocin, adrenocorticotropic hormone releasor and pituitary ACTH. Others are aldosterone-secretion regulator, thyroid-stimulating hormone (TSH) releasor, pituitary TSH, gonadotropins, growth hormone and lipid mobilizer.

The opinion prevails that the hypothalamus releases neurohumeral secretions that pass principally by way of the median eminence through portal veins. The secretions continue to the pars distalis of the adenohypophysis, releasing the pituitary tropic hormones. The hypothalamus is also believed to be a center for hormonal homeostasis resulting from a feed-back process.

CLINICAL FEATURES OF HYPOTHALAMIC TUMORS AND ADJACENT TUMORS INVADING OR COMPRESSING THE HYPOTHALAMUS.—Numerous neoplasms may involve the hypothalamus. These include craniopharyngioma, dermoid cyst and gliomas that arise in the optic chiasm, hypothalamus, third ventricle or midbrain. Meningioma, ectopic pinealoma, hamartoma of the tuber cinereum or mammillary bodies, lymphoma and metastatic neoplasms also involve this gland. These lesions produce symptoms of hypersomnia and somnolence, particularly if the posterior hypothalamus is involved. Narcolepsy and cataplexy are sometimes present. Invasion of the "satiety" centers, bilaterally, often leads to obesity from overeating; but, rarely, more laterally placed lesions may cause starvation. Increased thirst is common and is usually associated with diabetes insipidus. Slowly growing suprasellar tumors may produce pituitary insufficiency by blocking the portal circulation from the hypothalamus to the pars distalis. This may result in adrenocortical insufficiency, hypothyroidism, sexual precocity, hypogonadism or growth deficiency.

Sexual precocity.—This precocity may be defined as the onset of puberty before the age of 8 years in girls or 10 years in boys. It may result from lesions of the hypothalamus. In this instance, early secretion of gonadotropic hormones produces normal but precocious development and maturation of the gonads. Secretion of sex hormone is in the quantity of that in the normal adolescent or adult. This change is called complete sexual precocity. With tumors that involve the mammillary bodies or posterior hypothalamus, sexual precocity is more frequent. Tumors of the pineal body and quadrigeminal plates and hamartomas of the tuber cinereum have been found in many instances. Craniopharyngioma and tumors of the infundibulum and anterior hypothalamus often inhibit sexual maturation. Neoplasms of the optic chiasm, however, often produce precocious sexual development.

The sexual development is early but otherwise normal when precocity results from hypothalamic or pineal tumors. The prepubertal growth spurt is early and may precede development of the genitalia and secondary sex characteristics. Growth of the skeleton is accelerated more than is maturation, which leads to early closure of the epiphyses. Thus, although growth of the skeleton is initially accelerated, the bone length and body height are ultimately stunted. Dental development may be accelerated, but less than maturation and growth. After cessation of growth, most patients retain the bodily proportions of a child, with the head large and the extremities short compared to the trunk. The earlier the onset of the disease, the shorter the ultimate stature of the patient.

Excretion of neutral 17-ketosteroids and reducing corticoids is usually elevated for the patient's chronologic age but normal for the bone age. In some boys, an increased output of dehydroisoandosterone is found because of hyperfunction of the adrenal cortex. Estrogenic and androgenic hormones are present in the urine after the onset of puberty.

Hypothalamic neoplasms associated with precocity are from three to five times as common in boys as in girls, although the reverse is true for idiopathic sexual precocity. Sexual precocity from identifiable hypothalamic tumor is uncommon (probably less than 0.3%) compared to that from other lesions.

Retarded sexual development.—Sexual infantilism also may result from hypothalamic tumors. Growth of the patient may be stunted because of involvement of the anterior pituitary gland or its hypothalamic connections. Other patients may be of average height or tall, with eunuchoid proportions. Symptoms of hypothalamic involvement may be present. Froelich's syndrome (hypothalamic infantilism with obesity) is rare and is often confused with the more common benign syndrome of malfunctioning hypothalamus. It may result from a tumor or cyst in the vicinity of the hypothalamus or from a tumor of the pituitary gland encroaching on the brain. In the differentiation of these two types of "adiposogenital dystrophy," thyroid or adrenal insufficiency suggests organic disease, such as a neoplasm.

Dwarfism from hypothalamic tumors.—This type of dwarfism results, presumably, from lack of growth hormone secretion by the pituitary gland. Unless there are neurologic signs or metabolic abnormalities related to the hypothalamus, the etiology may be difficult to determine. The association of dwarfism and diabetes insipidus is evidence of an organic lesion of the pituitary or hypothalamic gland. After stunting becomes apparent, growth proceeds at a very slow rate. Skeletal maturation is delayed as well. Usually there is a complete failure of sexual development. The testes or ovaries remain small, and secondary sexual characteristics do not appear.

PATHOLOGIC FEATURES.—In addition to pineal tumors, many other tumors, may involve the hypothalamus. These include astrocytoma, ependymoma, neurofibroma, ganglioneuroma, infundibuloma, hamartoma of the tuber cinereum or mammillary bodies, craniopharyngioma and teratoma. Epidermoid cysts, dermoid, histiocytosis, leukemia, Hodgkin's disease, meningioma and metastatic neoplasm may also be responsible. We will discuss only a few.

Craniopharyngioma.—This tumor is the most common in the sellar or suprasellar region of children and adolescents. It is slow-growing and may not produce symptoms until late in life, but usually it does so before 40 years. In about half the patients, symptoms appear before age 15. Symptoms vary, depending on the direction of growth. Some of these are visual disturbance, diabetes insipidus, sexual infantilism, hypopituitary dwarfism, pituitary cachexia, somnolence and disturbance of temperature regulation. Others are papilledema, diplopia, hemiparesis, spasticity, tremor, rigidity and cerebellar ataxia. Rarely, sexual precocity develops instead of sexual infantilism. Surgical treatment of children with dwarfism accelerates growth and maturation, but the production of growth hormone, as now measured, may remain subnormal.

The tumor develops from remnants of the craniopharyngeal duct, which formed as a pocket from the roof of the buccal cavity. The ectodermal cells of the craniopharyngeal pouch may form cysts or tumors. The solid tumors are composed of columnar cells on a basement membrane resembling adamantinoma. Squamous cells with masses of cornified tissues are found within the tumor and may contain calcium. The lesions are usually suprasellar but may be within the sella.

Hamartoma of the tuber cinereum.—This lesion is uncommon and is about the size of a pea. Epilepsy or mental retardation is present in about half the patients, some of whom die suddenly. The masses are composed of cells resembling astrocytes, which sometimes invade adjacent areas. Tracts of nerve fibers lead from the hamartoma to the pituitary stalk. With modern pneumoencephalography, the small lesions may be identified. The tumor is usually associated with sexual precocity, which may begin in the first or second year of life (Fig. 118).

ROENTGEN FEATURES

PLAIN ROENTGENOGRAMS OF THE SKULL.—Tumors of the hypothalamus may produce increased intracranial pressure that presents roentgen changes similar to those described for pineal tumors. When the lesion begins in childhood and is of long duration, the size of the skull increases. The sella may be enlarged because of dilatation of the anterior part of the third ventricle which projects into the sella. In some instances, the enlarged sella may seem to be expanded; the appearance is similar to that produced by an intrasellar mass. Usually, the posterior clinoids and free margin of the dorsum are destroyed.

Craniopharyngiomas may produce a large sella turcica (Fig. 119). The solid craniopharyngioma may be situated predominantly within the sella and cause expansion of the sella. It differs from the more rapidly growing pituitary tumors because of the thickening and increased density of the sellar walls. With cystic craniopharyngiomas, which are mainly suprasellar, the sella is often elongated and shallow with small posterior clinoids and thin, sharp anterior clinoids. When the sella turcica is large, a persistent craniopharyngeal canal should suggest the diagnosis of craniopharyngioma.

Calcification.—Calcification is demonstrated in about 10% of gliomas (Fig. 125). The highest incidence of calcification (50%) is in the oligodendroglioma. Next in incidence is its presence in the astrocytomas (25%) and ependymomas. The calcification may be punctate, amorphous, trabecular or arborizing. Trabecular calcification is most characteristic of gliomas. The calcification may be minute or extensive and usually involves a small part of the neoplasm. It is more common in slow-growing tumors.

Craniopharyngioma is the most common suprasellar tumor to calcify. Calcium is identifiable in 55–75% of cases. The calcium is nodular when it involves solid portions of the tumor, which may be in the sella (Fig. 119), or curvilinear when the upper portion of a cystic mass, which is usually suprasellar, is involved. It may be mixed when both elements are present.

Gliomas of the optic chiasm and nerves cause sellar and optic foraminal changes (Figs. 122 and 123, *A*). The tumors are frequent in children and patients with neurofibromatosis. The foramen is enlarged in more than 75% of the children with glioma of one optic nerve. With glioma of the chiasm, this enlargement is present in two thirds of the children and may involve both optic foramina. The large foramina differ from those caused by other, more rapidly growing lesions in that their margins are intact without evidence of erosion. The cranial margin of the optic canal may be wider than the orbital margin. The intracranial optic gliomas also cause flattening or depression of the tuberculum sellae and chiasmatic groove, resulting in apparent lengthening of the sella (Fig. 123, *A*). The anterior clinoid on the affected side may be elevated and enlarged.

PNEUMOGRAPHY.—The hypothalamic tumor may fill in the lower part of the third ventricle and its superior part be outlined by gas (Figs. 120 and

121). An irregular superior border of the tumor almost always indicates a glioma. An extraventricular lesion usually creates a smooth upper border. The border of metastatic implants also may be smooth. In some instances, the tumor occludes or distorts only the optic or infundibular recesses. The third ventricle is displaced laterally if the tumor is eccentric. Tumors of the posterior hypothalamus bulge anteriorly, often occluding the aqueduct of Sylvius. The third ventricle then dilates, displacing the lamina terminalis forward and blunting the optic and infundibular recesses.

Pneumoencephalograms often show craniopharyngiomas to be in the interpeduncular cistern. Larger masses encroach on the anteroinferior aspect of the third ventricle. They obliterate the optic and infundibular recesses, presenting a mass whose curved surface is surrounded by air in the third ventricle. A sufficiently large mass occludes the foramen of Monro, produces hydrocephalus and projects into the anteroinferior surfaces of the lateral ventricles. The peduncles and aqueduct of Sylvius may be displaced posteriorly. The tumor may extend into the upper aspect of the pontine cistern.[7]

Glioma of the optic chiasm appears as a rounded mass surrounded by air above the tuberculum sellae near the optic groove (Figs. 123, B, and 125). These tumors impinge on the interpeduncular cistern and obliterate the chiasmatic cistern. The anteroinferior surface of the third ventricle is indented and displaced. A large tumor may obstruct the foramen of Monro, dilating the lateral ventricle.

Hamartoma of the tuber cinereum appears as a rounded, sharply delineated mass about the size of a pea and projects into the interpeduncular cistern (Fig. 118).

ANGIOGRAPHY.—Suprasellar tumors may be divided into anterior, middle and posterior lesions. The suprasellar lesion may displace the supraclinoid part of the carotid siphon upward and laterally. An elevation of the bifurcation of the internal carotid artery may be noted. The horizontal portion of the anterior cerebral artery may be displaced up and forward, and the proximal portion may be elevated. These changes may be present with suprasellar extension of a pituitary adenoma as well as with a primary suprasellar lesion. The carotid siphon may be displaced laterally along with the proximal anterior choroidal and posterior communicating arteries. Some large suprasellar tumors that block the foramen may elevate the internal cerebral vein.

The anterior suprasellar lesions in the region of the tuberculum sellae or planum sphenoidale are usually meningiomas and are seldom associated with endocrine disease.

Optic nerve gliomas may elevate the transverse part of the anterior cere-

---

[7] Epstein, *op. cit.*, 3.

bral artery and displace the internal carotid artery down and backward. Tumors of the optic chiasm displace the internal carotid, proximal posterior communicating and anterior choroidal arteries laterally (Fig. 124). Large tumors elevate the internal cerebral vein.

Posterior suprasellar masses produce lateral displacement of the anterior choroidal and posterior communicating arteries. They also displace the bifurcation of the internal carotid artery up and forward.

Even when a craniopharyngioma is large, angiograms may reveal few changes. Vascular staining of suprasellar gliomas or other tumors is uncommon.

SKELETAL ABNORMALITIES.—*Dwarfism* may result from deficiency of growth hormone or from premature closure of the epiphyses of the extremities or spine and be associated with sexual precocity. It may also result from other metabolic abnormalities. The bones of the pituitary hypothalamic dwarf continue to grow, but at a very slow rate. The appearance of the epiphyses is usually greatly delayed (Fig. 120), and their fusion may be delayed indefinitely or until adult life. Skeletal maturation and bone growth are both delayed (growth perhaps more so). Sexual development is totally absent. The lack of muscular development noted in adolescence persists. Skeletal proportions are normal, although the head may be large when hydrocephalus is present.

Sexual maturation may be delayed in patients who are not dwarfs or who may be tall with eunuchoid proportions. The adolescent spurt of growth and muscular development does not occur in these patients. The extremities are disproportionately long compared to the trunk. The length of the bones may be retarded at adolescence because of the lack of growth spurt. Because the epiphyseal cartilage persists, growth may continue into adult life, resulting in unusually long tubular bones. The changes of the skeleton caused by sex hormones are not seen in these patients.

Precocious sexual development.—Longitudinal bone growth is accelerated early and to a marked degree. Skeletal maturation demonstrated by appearance and fusion of epiphyses, occurs to an even greater extent than growth, so that the child may be tall initially but after premature fusion of the epiphyses stature is short. The body is characterized by short limbs, and the head is large.

Formation, eruption and size of the teeth are usually normal but may be minimally accelerated. With shortening of the jaw from early growth failure, the teeth may be crowded.

Figure 112.—Pineal tumor.

A, posteroanterior projection, revealing pineal calcification (**arrow**) lying to the left of the midline.

B (same patient as in *A*), pneumoencephalogram, demonstrating a large round soft tissue mass (**a**) within which lies the eccentrically placed calcific debris (**arrow**) noted in *A*. The foramen of Monro is seen at **b**; the suprapineal recess at **c**; moderately dilated third ventricle at **d**; incompletely filled lateral ventricle at **e**, and the temporal horn at **f**.

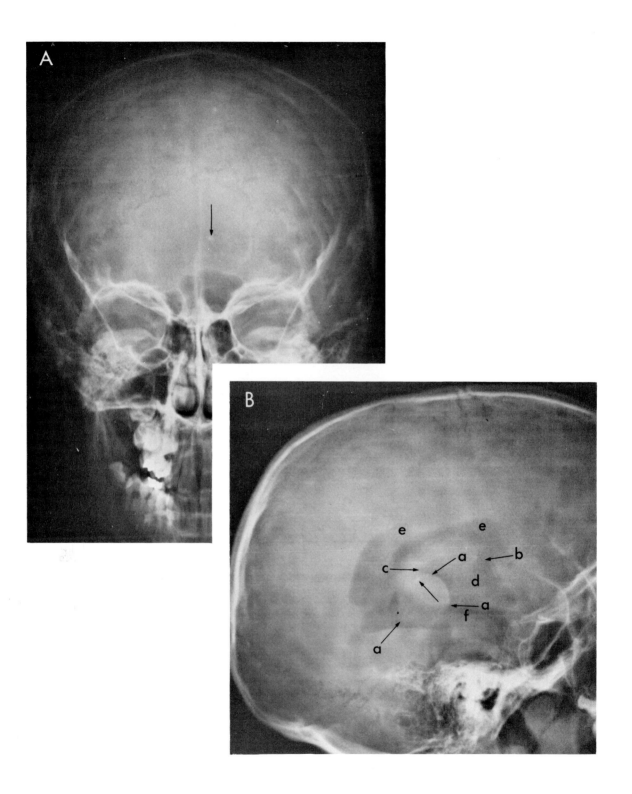

Figure 112 · Pineal Tumor: Calcification / 301

Figure 113.—Pineal tumor.

Lateral pneumoencephalogram, revealing pronounced dilatation of the lateral ventricles (**a**). The third ventricle (**b**) is dilated, displaced anteriorly and encroached upon by a very large pineal tumor (**c**), which also has displaced the sylvian aqueduct anteriorly (**d**). Note the asymmetrically placed, greatly enlarged calcification (**arrow**) within the tumor.

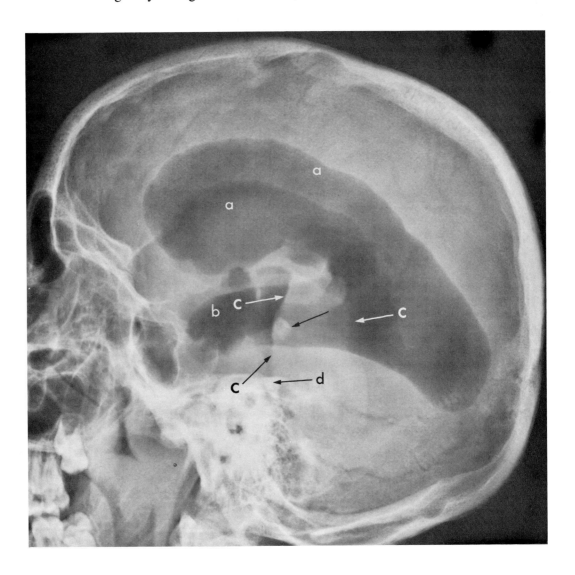

Figure 114.—Pineal tumor.

Fractional lateral pneumoencephalogram: a large pineal tumor (**a**) encroaches on the third ventricle (**b**). Note the very small deposit of calcific debris within the tumor (**arrow**).

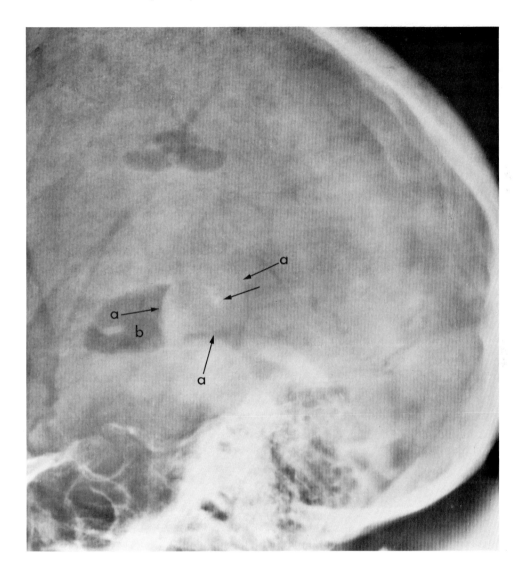

Figure 114 · Pineal Tumor: Calcification / 303

Figure 115.—Pineal tumor.

Posteroanterior body-section radiograph, demonstrating the "cut-off" (**arrow**) of the rostral end of the moderately dilated third ventricle (**x**). Note the normal floor of the sella turcica.

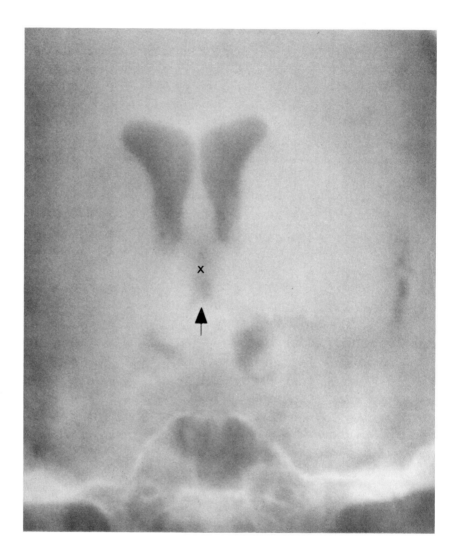

Figure 116.—Ectopic pineal tumor.

Midline lateral tomogram, revealing extension of a pineal tumor (**arrows**) along the floor of the third ventricle, which is encroached upon (**a**). Note the dilated anterior horn of the lateral ventricle (**x**).

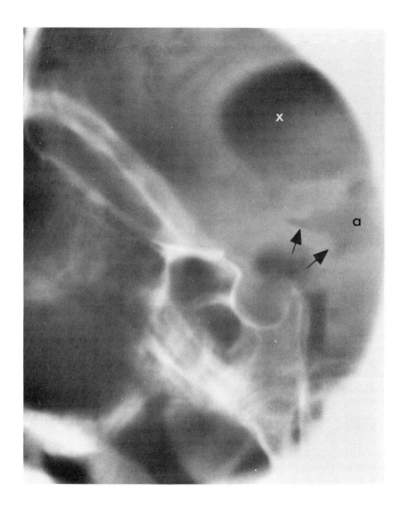

Figure 116 · **Ectopic Pineal Tumor** / **305**

Figure 117.—Ectopic pinealoma.

Midline tomogram of the lateral pneumoencephalogram: A large ectopic pineal tumor (**arrows**) encroaches on the anterior aspect of the third ventricle (**a**). The lateral ventricles are not dilated.

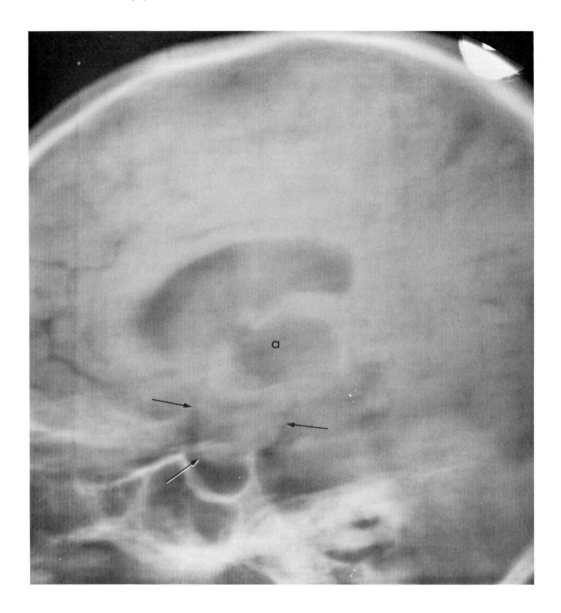

Figure 118.—Hamartoma of the tuber cinereum.

Midline tomogram of a lateral ventriculogram: A large soft tissue tumor (**x**) lies immediately above and behind the dorsum sellae (**arrow**), obliterating the cisterna interpeduncularis. The third ventricle (**a**) is partially demonstrated. The fourth ventricle (**b**) and quadrigeminal plate (**c**) are beautifully delineated. The optic chiasm (**d**) is seen with ease. Somewhat less distinct is the stalk of the pituitary (**e**). The air-filled sphenoid sinus lies at **f**.

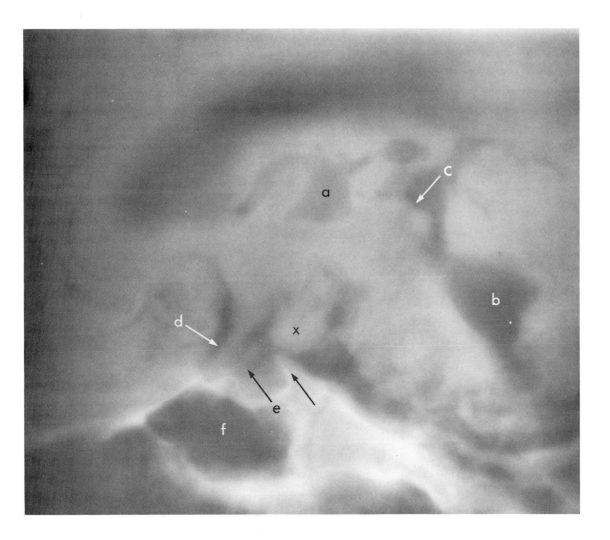

Figure 118 · Hamartoma of the Tuber Cinereum / 307

Figure 119.—Probable craniopharyngioma.

A, lateral roentgenogram of the skull of a 34-year-old man with short stature. The sella turcica is enlarged, with backward displacement of the dorsum sellae. A calcific density is present anterior to it. The lesion was not explored but was probably a craniopharyngioma.

B (same patient as in *A*), posteroanterior view of the right hand. The secondary ossification centers of the proximal phalanges and the distal ends of the radius and ulna are unfused. The degree of bone maturation is consistent with that of a normal 16-year-old. Sexual development in this patient was retarded and was associated with short stature. Some patients with retarded maturation have normal secretion of growth hormone and normal stature.

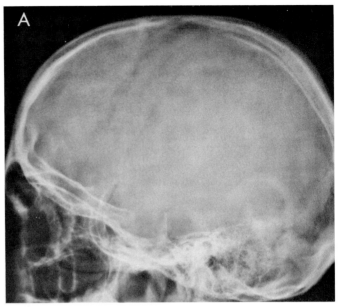

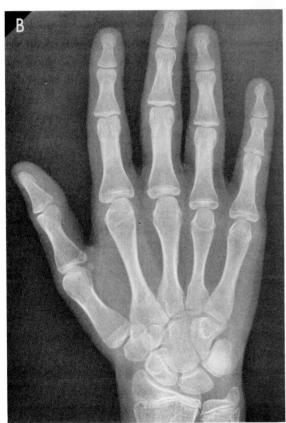

Figure 119 · Probable Craniopharyngioma / 309

Figure 120.—Hypothalamic glioma with pronounced delayed bone development (all figures from same patient).

A, lateral brow-up pneumoencephalogram of a 4-year-old child, showing marked lateral ventricular dilatation and almost complete obliteration of the third ventricle. The sella is enlarged.

B, pneumoencephalogram, revealing evidence of lateral ventricular dilatation, which is symmetrical. The third ventricle has not been demonstrated.

C, posteroanterior roentgenogram of the hand, demonstrating bone age of approximately 1 year, in contrast to the chronologic age of 4.

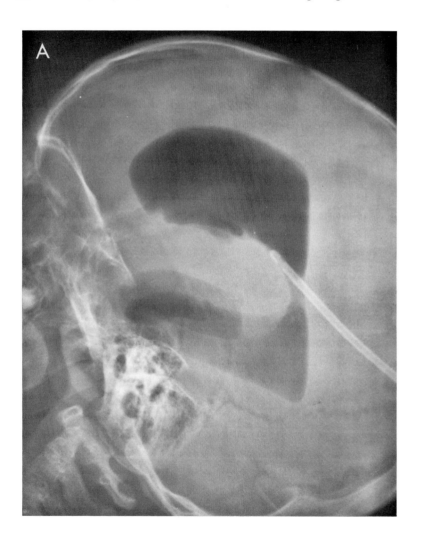

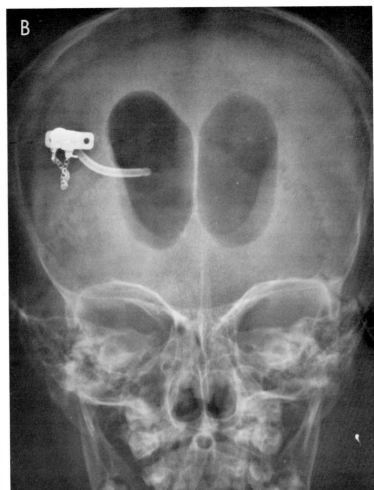

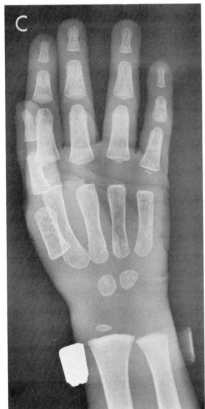

Figure 120 · Hypothalamic Glioma / 311

Figure 121.—Hypothalamic glioma.

A, lateral brow-up midline body-section radiograph of a pneumoencephalogram, revealing a tumor (**x**) invading the hypothalamic portion of the third ventricle (**a**). The foramen of Monro (**b**), lateral ventricle (**c**) and the cisterna ponti (**d**) are clearly seen.

B (same patient as in *A*), anteroposterior arteriogram, demonstrating elevation of the anterior cerebral artery (**arrow**).

This patient showed evidence of delayed sexual maturation.

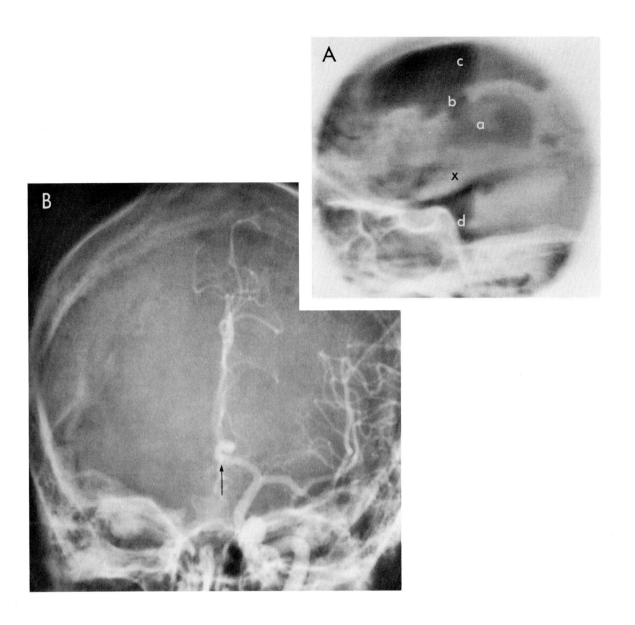

Figure 121 · Hypothalamic Glioma / 313

Figure 122.—Glioma of the optic chiasm.

Views of right (**A**) and left (**B**) optic foramina, delineating bilateral enlargement secondary to a glioma of the optic chiasm (**arrow**). The cortical margins of the foramina are intact and of normal thickness because of the neoplasm's slow growth.

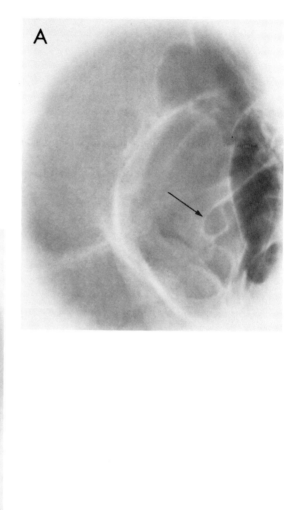

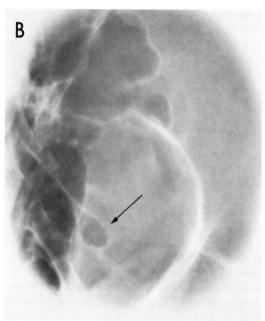

Figure 122 · Glioma of the Optic Chiasm / 315

Figure 123.—Gliomas of the optic chiasm.

A, routine lateral roentgenogram of the skull: Marked erosion and elongation of the chiasmatic sulcus (**a**) are seen, as well as erosion of the anterior clinoids (**b**). There is some widening of the sutures due to increased intracranial pressure.

B, lateral projection of a pneumoencephalogram of another patient: A tumor of the optic chiasm (**x**) obliterates the cisterna chiasmaticus and extends partially into the cisterna interpeduncularis.

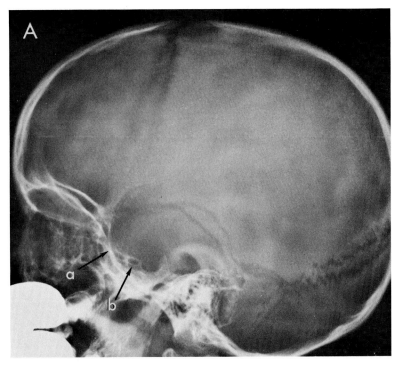

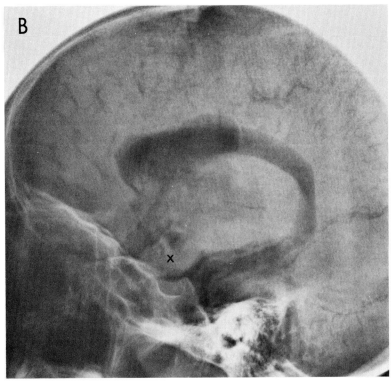

Figure 123 · Glioma of the Optic Chiasm / 317

Figure 124.—Glioma of the optic chiasm.

A, lateral arteriogram: Marked bowing and stretching of the anterior cerebral artery (**arrows**) caused by a mass arising in the optic chiasm.

B (same patient as in *A*), anteroposterior arteriogram: Pronounced lateral displacement of the anterior cerebral artery (**arrow**) and similar but minor displacement of the internal carotid artery (**a**) above the carotid siphon.

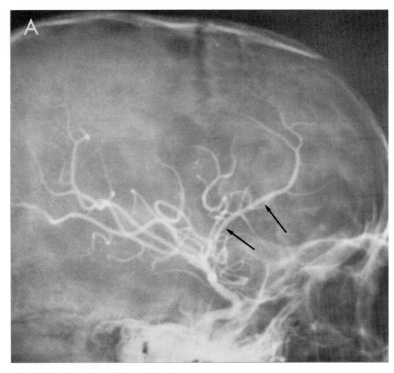

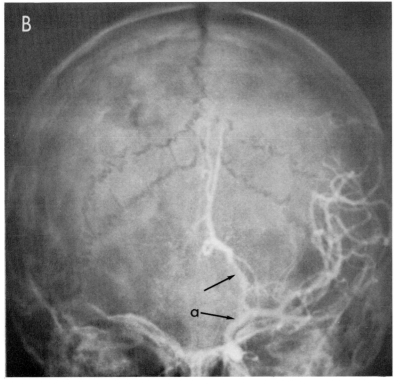

Figure 124 · Glioma of the Optic Chiasm / 319

Figure 125.—Glioma of the optic chiasm.

A, lateral pneumoencephalogram: A huge mass (**x**) outlined by air (**arrows**) occupies the chiasmatic and interpeduncular cisterns.

B (same patient as in *A*), lateral projection 3 years later, following craniotomy. Calcific debris presumably lying within the residual tumor is faintly demonstrated (**arrows**). There is no evidence of increased intracranial pressure.

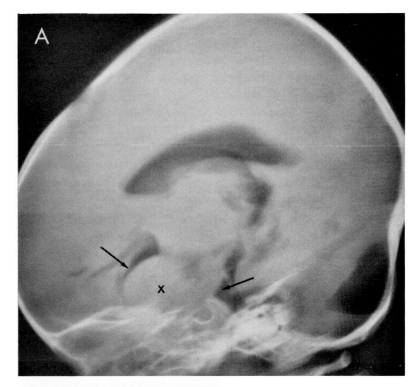

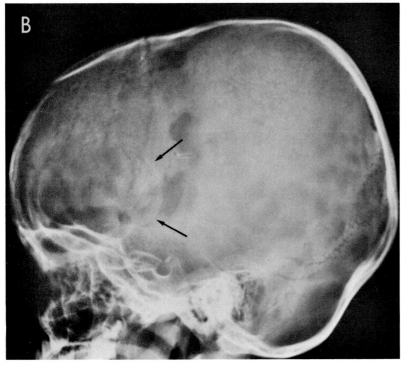

Figure 125 · Glioma of the Optic Chiasm / 321

Index

HYPOTELORISM, with neuroblastoma, 214–15
HYPOTHALAMUS, 293 ff.
    anatomy, 293
    function, 293 f.
    invasion or compression by adjacent tumors, 294
    tumors, 294 ff.
        clinical features, 294 ff.
        dwarfism with, 295, 296
        pathology, 296
        roentgen study
        —angiography, 298, 312, 318–19
        —pneumoencephalography, 297 f., 307–13, 316–17, 320–21
        —skull studies, 296 f., 307–21
        sexual infantilism with, 295
        sexual precocity with, 294

I

ILIUM, in hyperparathyroidism, 88
INSULINOMA, 152–53
ISCHIUM, in hyperparathyroidism, 88, 108–109

J

JOINTS, in acromegaly, 6, 28–31

K

KIDNEY INVOLVEMENT
    by adrenal tumors, 161, 174–77, 182–83, 188–91, 194–99, 203, 205, 230–31
    by neuroblastoma, 167, 203, 205, 207, 214
    by pancreatic sarcoma, 142–43
    by pheochromocytoma, 218–21, 224–29
    by testicular tumors, 275, 277, 284–85
KNEE: in hyperparathyroidism, 89, 112–13

L

LEIOMYOSARCOMA TESTIS, 284–85
LITHIASIS, PANCREATIC, with pseudocysts, 124

LIVER METASTASES
    from neuroblastoma, 167, 210–15
    from pancreatic tumor, 140–41
LUNG METASTASES
    from testicular tumors, 267, 274–75, 282–83
    from thyroid, 44, 48, 66–69
LYMPH NODE METASTASES
    from testicular tumors, 266 f., 274–75
    from thyroid carcinoma, 43, 44, 64–65
LYMPHANGIOGRAPHY, for testicular tumor metastases, 267
LYMPHOMA, THYROID, 45, 56–57

M

MANDIBLE, in acromegaly, 6, 7, 26–27
MASTOID(S), in acromegaly, 7, 24–25
MAXILLA, in hyperparathyroidism, 104–105
MEDIASTINUM
    goiter in, 50–51, 54–59
    metastases
        from neuroblastoma, 169
        from pheochromocytoma, 234–35
    parathyroid neoplasms in, 94–97
MEIGS' SYNDROME, 241, 260–61
MYELOLIPOMA(S), ADRENAL, 158

N

NEPHROCALCINOSIS, in hyperparathyroidism, 88, 98–99
NEUROBLASTOMA(S)
    abdominal vs. intrathoracic, 167
    calcification in, 167, 202–205, 212–13
    metastases, 166, 167
        to liver, 202–205, 212–13
        skeletal, 168, 212–17
    of organ of Zuckerkandl, 170, 209, 210
    pelvic, 208–209
    roentgen study, 167 f., 202–15

O

ORGAN OF ZUCKERKANDL, neuroblastoma of, 170, 209, 210

THYROID (*cont.*)
    adenocarcinoma—metastases, 43, 48, 64–69
    follicular, 43 f., 52–53
    —metastases, 44, 48, 68, 70–75
    giant cell, 45
    Hürtle cell, 44 f.
    medullary, 44, 54–55
    metastases, 43, 44, 45, 48 f., 64–77
    papillary, 43
    —in benign adenoma, 62–63
    —calcification in, 62–63
    —in thyroglossal duct cyst, 60, 61
    solid, 44
    spindle cell, 45
    with Zollinger-Ellison syndrome, 138
  diseases, 39 ff.
    neck mass, 45 f.
    roentgen changes, 45 ff.
  lingual, 47, 60
  lymphoma, 45, 56–57
  malignant tumors, 43 ff.
    arteriography in, 48, 64–65
    calcification in, 43, 47, 60–63
    differentiation from goiter, 48
    metastases, 43, 44, 45, 48 f., 64–65
    roentgen characteristics, 46 f., 52–55
  tumors, vis-à-vis parathyroid tumors, 89
TIBIA
  in hyperparathyroidism, 88, 106–107
  neuroblastoma metastases, 212–13
TOES
  clubbing, in thyroid acropachy, 45
  subperiosteal resorption in hyperparathyroidism, 102–103
TRACHEA
  with mediastinal goiter, 47, 58–59
  with nodular goiter, 46, 50–51, 58–59
  with parathyroid tumor, 92–93

  with thyroid carcinoma, 52–55, 66–67
  with thyroid lymphosarcoma, 56–57

U

ULCER (GASTRODUODENAL), with Zollinger-Ellison syndrome, 121, 132–33
URINARY TRACT, in hyperparathyroidism, 85 f., 88, 98–99

V

VENA CAVA, with seminoma testis, 278–79
VENTRICLES
  with hypothalamic lesions, 297 f., 307–308, 312–13
  with pineal tumors, 292, 300–306
VERTEBRAE
  in acromegaly, 7, 34–35
  in Cushing's syndrome, 162, 184–85, 192–93, 200–201
  metastases from thyroid, 76–77
  in secondary hyperparathyroidism, 90

W

WRIST
  with adrenal adenoma, 176–77
  chondrocalcinosis in, 110, 111

Z

ZOLLINGER-ELLISON SYNDROME
  endocrine tumors with, 121
  metastases, 138–41
  non-beta islet cell tumors with, 120
  pathology, 120
  roentgen findings, 121, 132–41
    tumor blush, 122, 136–37, 152–53
  ulcer diathesis with, 121, 132–33